A Manual of Clinical Laparoscopy

GYNECOLOGICAL ENDOSCOPY MANUAL SERIES

A Manual of Clinical Laparoscopy

Michael P. Diamond, MD

Director, Division of Reproductive Endocrinology and Infertility
Professor, Departments of Obstetrics and Gynecology, and Physiology
Wayne State University, Detroit, MI, USA

Foreword by

Alan H. DeCherney, MD

Professor and Chairman, Department of Obstetrics and Gynecology
University of California, Los Angeles School of Medicine
Los Angeles, CA, USA

The Parthenon Publishing Group
International Publishers in Medicine, Science & Technology

NEW YORK   LONDON

Library of Congress Cataloging-in-Publication Data
Diamond, Michael P.
    A manual of clinical laparoscopy / Michael P. Diamond.
       p.   cm. -- (Gynecological endoscopy manual series)
    Includes bibliographical references and index.
    ISBN 1-85070-640-9
    1. Generative organs, Female--Endoscopic surgery.
2. Laparoscopy.   3. Generative organs, Female--Diseases--
Diagnosis. I. Title. II. Series.
    [DNLM: 1. Genital Diseases, Female--surgery--handbooks.
2. Genital Diseases, Female--diagnosis--handbooks. 3. Surgery,
Laparoscopic--handbooks. 4. Laparoscopy--handbooks.
WP 39 D537m 1997]
RG104.7.D535 1997
618.1'059--dc21
DNLM/DLC
for Library of Congress   97-18021
                                    CIP

British Library Cataloguing in Publication Data
Diamond, Michael P.
    A manual of clinical laparoscopy. - (Gynecological endoscopy
manual series)
    1. Laparoscopy - Handbooks, manuals, etc. 2. Generative
organs, Female - Diseases - Diagnosis - Handbooks, manuals, etc.
I. Title
618.1'07545

    ISBN 1-85070-640-9

Published in the USA by
The Parthenon Publishing Group Inc.
One Blue Hill Plaza
PO Box 1564, Pearl River
New York 10965, USA

Published in the UK and Europe by
The Parthenon Publishing Group Limited
Casterton Hall, Carnforth
Lancs. LA6 2LA, UK

Copyright ©1998
Parthenon Publishing Group

Printed and bound in Spain by
T.G. Hostench, S.A.

Contents

Foreword

Michael Diamond has written an extremely important contribution to the surgical literature in the form of *A Manual of Clinical Laparoscopy*. Not only does this text cover the basics of anatomy, instrumentation and other surgical tools, but a 'how-to' section has also been included.

The author has reviewed specific disease entities and illustrated each chapter in a professional, concise and comprehensive manner. Many surgeons who perform endoscopic surgery learn this skill as their only mode of therapy; they also consider that the basics, which are of tantamount importance to those surgeons who carry out open surgery, do not carry the same intellectual urgency when involving the use of endoscopy. This is not true and, with this manual, the author has provided the basic information required in this important area of expertise for the optimal performance of endoscopic surgery.

The same can be said of the instrumentation used in endoscopy. It is possibly true that, to quote a well-known phrase, it is not necessary to know how a car works in order to drive it. However, most would agree that we would be better drivers if we at least had some understanding of how a car works. The same could be said of the instrumentation used for laparoscopic surgery. It is not necessary to understand the principle of the Hopkins lens, but it is important to know the diameters of the instruments and the power source as well as to have a facility with the various instruments available to achieve the best results in terms of both safety and efficiency for a given situation. Through this manual, Dr Diamond has provided us with the intellectual 'aces' and tools for laparoscopic surgery.

Many novice surgeons, when queried as to why they do what they do, are unable to answer. I consider this to be a genuine problem and an offshoot of the burgeoning use of the laparoscope in gynecological surgery. It has become, for whatever reason, somehow acceptable to not have an explanation for the procedures and techniques used in laparoscopy compared with the rationales behind open surgical procedures. This may perhaps simply be a 'sign of the times' as regards criticism, or it may be that minimally invasive surgery is being mistaken for minimally informative surgery!

The 'how-to' section of this manual is superb and even covers to the finest detail the optimal preparation of the operating room for laparoscopic surgery. Thus, this manual answers the question that I am so frequently asked: How should I set up my operating room to perform laparoscopic surgery?

Each of the pathological entities, such as ectopic pregnancy, myomectomy and adhesiolysis, are handled comprehensively and with great skill, and with a minimum of repetition. Areas of controversy, such as the use of laparoscopy for myomectomy, are well addressed. Peppered throughout the text are useful tips, such as the 'classical tenets of gynecological microsurgery' listed in the adhesiolysis chapter which, in fact, apply techniques from open procedures.

In an encyclopedic way, yet providing all of the necessary information in one text, this manual addresses both the more common procedures, such as those for ectopic pregnancy, as well as those that are more esoteric, such as the treatment of stress incontinence and other pelvic floor defects, performed via the laparoscope. The book closes with a helpful chapter on anesthesia and a selected bibliography that includes the classics on the subject.

This is a work that is itself destined to become a classic in that it is the first stand-alone manual for laparoscopy and, as laparoscopy becomes more important, so will this book. The author is a fine educator who writes well and, because of his preciseness, has given us a very useful text. Neither has Dr Diamond shied away from controversy as, even in such a concise manual as this, areas that are still under discussion are not just simply swept under the carpet. This book is indeed the work of a well-trained practitioner and constitutes an important contribution to the currently available literature in this field.

Alan H. DeCherney, MD
Los Angeles

Preface

Learning to perform surgery is a continuing process of education. Although a student can achieve a great deal by reading, observing videotaped procedures and live surgery, and participating in training and post-graduate courses as well as by practicing on inanimate and animate models, none of these approaches can replace first-hand clinical experience in the operating room.

I have been extremely fortunate to have had the opportunity to undergo a large part of my training under the guidance of a number of surgeons while attending Vanderbilt University in Nashville, TN and Yale University in New Haven, CT. I am particularly indebted to Drs James F. Daniell and Alan H. DeCherney for their surgical teaching and the opportunities they have provided me. However, it would be remiss not to also acknowledge my gratitude to Drs Lonnie S. Burnett, Howard Jones III, Stephen Entman, Wayne Maxson, Mary Lake Polan and Stephen Boyers. Finally, I am especially grateful to my colleague D. Alan Johns, who

has kindly provided a number of the surgical photographs included in this book.

As no discussion of laparoscopic surgery would be complete without an introduction to anesthesia, I am grateful to Drs Raymond Glassenberg and Samuel Glassenberg for their in-depth consideration of the art of laparoscopic anesthesia for inclusion in this book. In addition, I wish to thank Drs Ceana Nezhat, Farr Nezhat and Camran Nezhat for their contribution on the newer laparoscopic treatments of stress incontinence and other pelvic floor defects, which completes the range of techniques covered in this volume. Furthermore, I am grateful to Sharyn Wong of Parthenon Publishing, who has been very helpful in the production of this book.

Finally, I would like to thank my wife Meredith, and my children Samantha, Ryan, Matthew, Justin and Brendan, for allowing me to take precious time away from my family obligations to write this book.

Michael P. Diamond
Detroit

Introduction

This manual of laparoscopy is intended to be a basic primer on the performance of laparoscopy, and is primarily aimed at the junior resident, intern and medical student. The intention of this book is to provide information not only on what to do and how to do it, but also why. The latter is of particular importance because, in surgery, every patient is unique and, although there may be similarities to previous cases, new situations always arise. To only know what and how without knowing why may potentially lead to a situation in which the practitioner will be inadequately prepared to deal with a sudden turn of events, with the possible result that the patient's therapy may be less efficient, less complete or accompanied by complications. Without a knowledge and understanding of the basic principles of laparoscopic surgery, the lack of an appreciation of why is even more likely to occur.

The ideas expressed in this manual include opinions for which no well-established data are available. Therefore, others may find that there are equally acceptable or possibly better ways to accomplish the same goals. Furthermore, as with most areas of clinical medicine, there are exceptions to every rule, and new advances continue to be made that may lead to refinements and alterations to previously accepted practices. Thus, any principles and procedures must be appropriately modified to take into account the particulars of the patient, operating theater, surgeon's experience, available personnel, equipment and instruments.

Familiarity with the concepts in this volume should be viewed as only the initial step towards becoming an endoscopic surgeon. Further expertise and experience need to be acquired through other activities such as attending lectures and courses, practicing with inanimate objects, tissue and animals, assisting an experienced endoscopic surgeon and practicing while being observed by an experienced surgeon.

Finally, it is beyond the scope of this book to cover all aspects of the relevant topics in depth, such as patient selection, preoperative management and advanced procedures. For further reading on the subject, the reader is referred to the sources listed in the selected bibliography.

1 Anatomy of the pelvis

Abdominal wall

The abdominal wall is composed of seven layers (Figure 1.1). The outermost layer is the skin and immediately beneath the skin is the subcutaneous fascia, which is generally divided into a superficial fatty layer (Camper's fascia) and a deeper elastic layer (Scarpa's fascia). The thickness of the subcutaneous fat layer varies greatly according to a person's weight and body fat distribution. Scarpa's fascia in the vicinity of the umbilicus is usually extremely thin and often cannot be appreciated tactually when traversed by a Veress needle or trocar.

Beneath Scarpa's fascia is another layer of fascia, the deep fascia, and a layer of muscle containing the rectus, external oblique, internal oblique and transversus abdominis muscles and their aponeuroses. The thickness of this layer and the relationships of the muscles to each other depend on both the coronal (Figure 1.2) and sagittal planes chosen. In the midline, the aponeuroses of all of these muscles are fused as the linea alba.

Proceeding laterally in either direction, the aponeuroses envelop the rectus muscles which originate from the ribs and extend to the pelvic brim. The aponeurosis of the internal oblique muscle is initially superficial to the rectus muscle at the level of the pubic symphysis, but splits approximately halfway between the umbilicus and pubic symphysis. Once lateral to the rectus muscle, the external oblique, internal oblique and transversus muscles can then be identified as continuations of their respective aponeuroses.

Deep to the muscle layer is a layer of preperitoneal fat and fibroelastic connective tissue followed by the final layer, the peritoneum. The peritoneal layer and the aponeurotic layer superficial to it are the two layers that are generally identifiable during placement of the Veress needle or trocar.

The thinnest segment of the abdominal wall is at the umbilicus, where many of these layers are fused together (Figure 1.3). The umbilicus usually overlaps the fourth lumbar (L4) vertebra and lies at the level of the aortic bifurcation (Figure 1.4). Thus, placement of the Veress needle or trocar at this site should not be perpendicular to the skin (which would cause the tip to point approximately at the bifurcation), but at an approximately 45° angle to the hollow of the pelvis.

Pelvis

The pelvis is a ring-like structure derived from the fusion of four bony segments: the two hip bones (comprising ilium, pubis and ischium), sacrum and coccyx (Figure 1.5). The adult pelvis can be subdivided into two components: the false (greater) pelvis; and the true (lesser) pelvis, which are adjacent to each other (Figure 1.6). The pubic symphysis is the junction of the two hip bones in the midline; of the abdominal wall muscles, the insertion of rectus abdominis lies closest to this junction (see Figure 1.5).

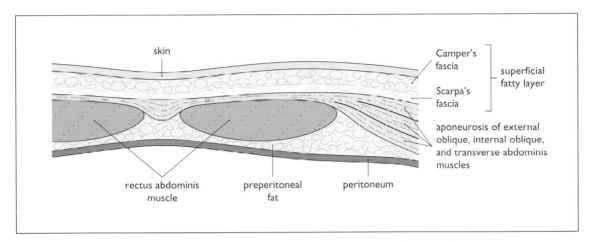

Figure 1.1 Transverse section through the anterior abdominal wall showing the seven layers that comprise its thickness

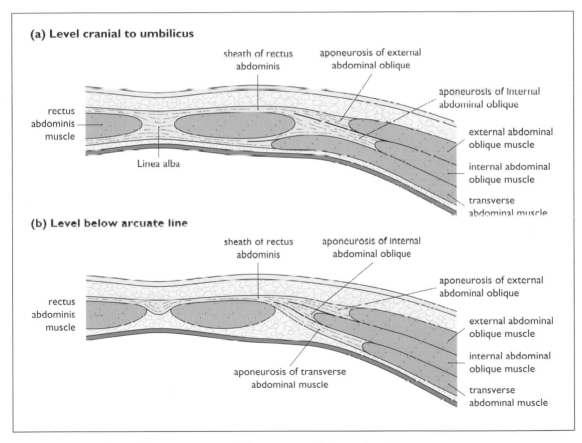

Figure 1.2 Transverse sections through the anterior abdominal wall at the level of the umbilicus (upper) and below the arcuate line (lower) show the differences in the thickness and relationship of the muscles and their aponeuroses

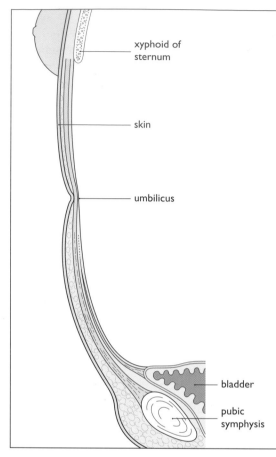

Figure 1.3 Longitudinal section through the anterior abdominal wall in the line of the umbilicus shows thinning at that point

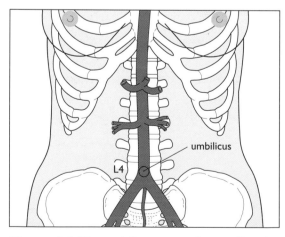

Figure 1.4 The umbilicus normally overlies the fourth lumbar vertebra at the level of the aortic bifurcation

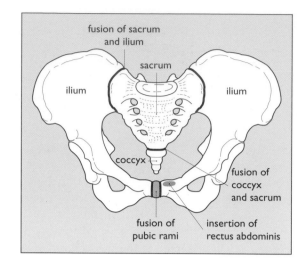

Figure 1.5 The pelvic girdle is derived from fusion of the two hip bones with the sacrum and the sacrum with the coccyx

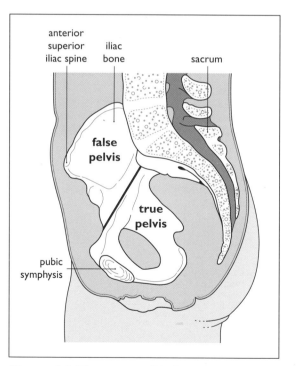

Figure 1.6 The greater (false) pelvis consists of the 'wings' of the iliac part of the hip bone above the linea terminalis on each side, and the base of the sacrum posteriorly. The lesser (true) pelvis is the narrowed continuation of the greater pelvis and encloses the pelvic cavity, which is of greatest obstetric importance

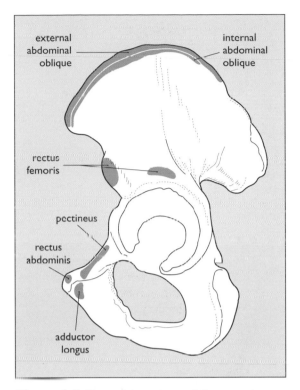

Figure 1.7 Sites of insertion of the muscles on the bony pelvis

Continuing laterally, the wings of the ilium form the insertion of the internal and external oblique muscles as well as many of the muscles of the pelvis and lower extremities (Figure 1.7). Caudally, the sacrum has multiple openings for the passage of vessels and nerve fibers to supply the legs, as well as the pelvis and perineum (Figure 1.8).

Blood supply

The arterial blood supply of the pelvis is derived from the descending aorta, which divides at approximately the level of L4 to form the right and left common iliac arteries and, often, a small branch which extends over the sacral promontory as the middle sacral artery (Figure 1.9). Each common iliac artery is approximately 5 cm long, and divides into external and internal iliac arteries.

The external iliac artery passes over the internal obturator muscle to exit the pelvis.

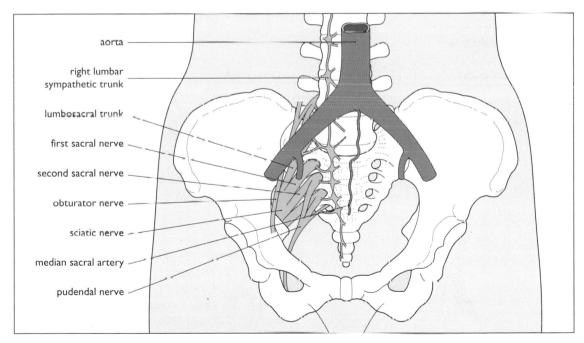

Figure 1.8 Right sacral plexus and right pelvic portion of the lumbar sympathetic trunk shown in relation to the abdominal aortic bifurcation and median sacral artery

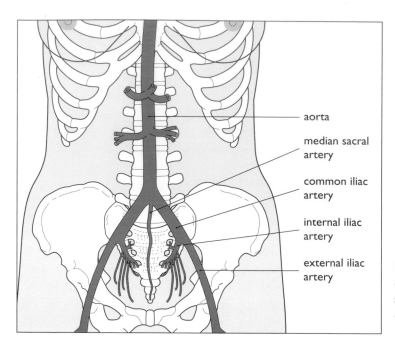

aorta

median sacral artery

common iliac artery

internal iliac artery

external iliac artery

Figure 1.9 Pelvic arterial supply derived from the common iliac arteries which branch from the descending aorta

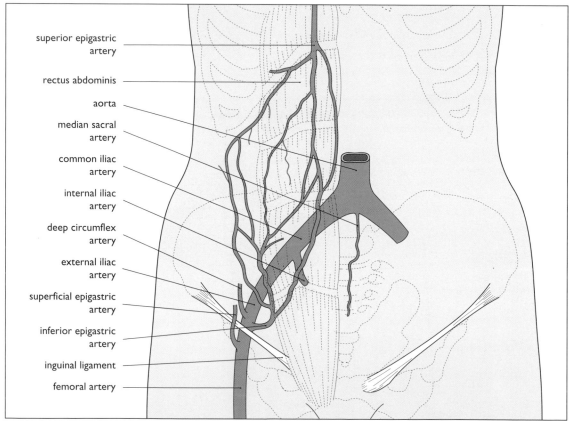

superior epigastric artery

rectus abdominis

aorta

median sacral artery

common iliac artery

internal iliac artery

deep circumflex artery

external iliac artery

superficial epigastric artery

inferior epigastric artery

inguinal ligament

femoral artery

Figure 1.10 The inferior epigastric artery, a branch of the external iliac, has important laparoscopic implications

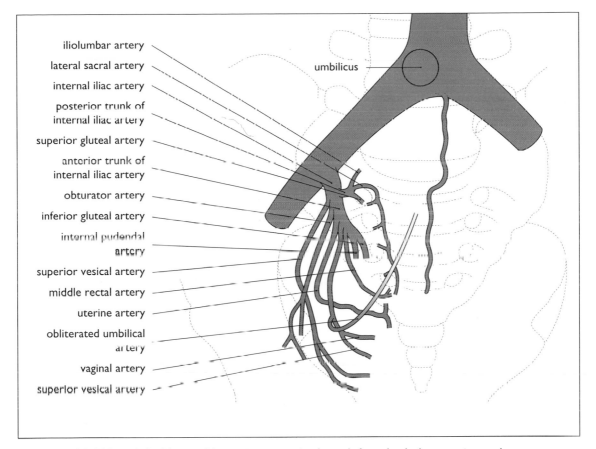

iliolumbar artery
lateral sacral artery
internal iliac artery
posterior trunk of internal iliac artery
superior gluteal artery
anterior trunk of internal iliac artery
obturator artery
inferior gluteal artery
internal pudendal artery
superior vesical artery
middle rectal artery
uterine artery
obliterated umbilical artery
vaginal artery
superior vesical artery

umbilicus

Figure 1.11 Although highly variable, various arteries branch from both the anterior and posterior trunks of the internal iliac artery

The external iliac usually has two branches, the inferior epigastric and the deep circumflex arteries (Figure 1.10). The inferior epigastric artery is especially important for laparoscopic surgeons because it is difficult to localize at the time of secondary trocar placement. The vessel arises immediately above the inguinal ligament and then curves ventrally to run essentially in parallel to the rectus abdominis; its terminal branches anastomose with branches of the superior epigastric and lower intercostal arteries (see Figure 1.10).

The internal iliac artery follows a path along the side wall of the pelvis towards the greater sciatic foramen. Although highly variable, along this path the internal iliac may give origin to a number of pelvic vessels (Figure 1.11) including: a posterior trunk, which often gives origin to the inferior gluteal and internal pudendal arteries; an anterior trunk, which often gives rise to the obliterated umbilical artery (an embryonic remnant that runs alongside the bladder towards the umbilicus) as well as visceral (superior and inferior vesical, middle rectal and uterine arteries) and musculoskeletal (internal pudendal, obturator, iliolumbar, lateral sacral and superior gluteal arteries) branches. Running alongside these arteries are the venous companions; the exception is the ovarian vein that drains into the inferior vena cava on the right and renal vein on the left (Figure 1.12).

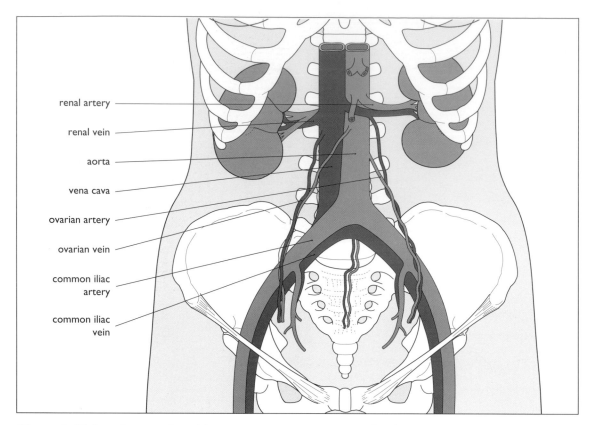

renal artery

renal vein

aorta

vena cava

ovarian artery

ovarian vein

common iliac artery

common iliac vein

Figure 1.12 Arteries run alongside venous companions except for the ovarian vein

Lymphatic supply

Drainage of the pelvic viscera into the pelvic lymphatic chains is variable (Figure 1.13); the more common patterns of drainage are listed in Table 1.1.

Nerve supply

The neural supply of interest to the gynecological laparoscopist arises primarily from the thoracic, lumbar, sacral and coccygeal portions of the spinal cord (Figure 1.14). The abdominal wall is innervated by the thoracic and lumbar nerves, in particular, from the seventh to eleventh thoracic nerves (Figure 1.15). The anterior divisions of these nerves generally circumscribe the body and run ventrally between the internal oblique

Table 1.1 Common lymphatic drainage of pelvic structures

Bladder
  external iliac nodes
  internal, external and common iliac nodes
  lateral vesical nodes
Ureter
  lateral aortic nodes
  common iliac nodes
  internal iliac nodes
Urethra
  internal iliac nodes
Ovary
  lateral and preaortic nodes
Uterine cervix
  internal, external and common iliac nodes
Uterine body and fundus
  lateral and preaortic nodes
Fallopian tube
  lateral and preaortic nodes
Vagina
  internal, external and common iliac nodes
  superficial inguinal nodes

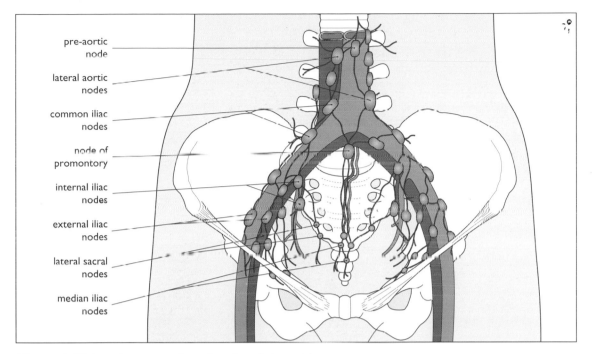

Figure 1.13 Lymphatic vessels and nodes of the pelvis

pre-aortic node

lateral aortic nodes

common iliac nodes

node of promontory

internal iliac nodes

external iliac nodes

lateral sacral nodes

median iliac nodes

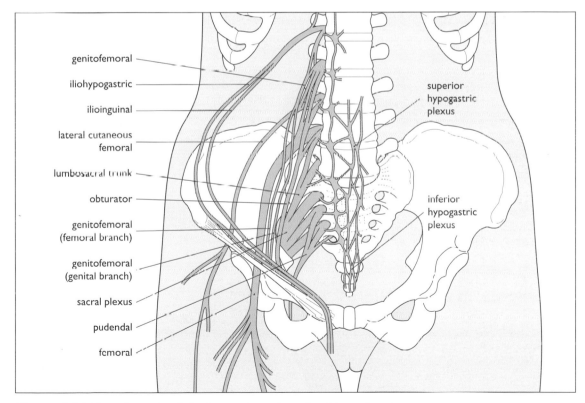

Figure 1.14 Neural supply of the lower thoracic and pelvic regions

genitofemoral

iliohypogastric

ilioinguinal

lateral cutaneous femoral

lumbosacral trunk

obturator

genitofemoral (femoral branch)

genitofemoral (genital branch)

sacral plexus

pudendal

femoral

superior hypogastric plexus

inferior hypogastric plexus

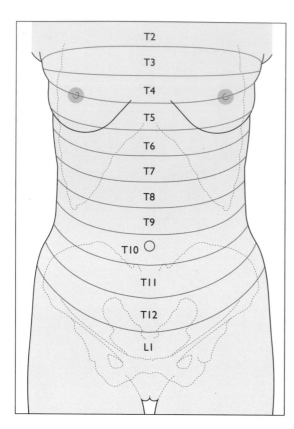

Figure 1.15 Approximate segmental distribution of the cutaneous nerves of the trunk are derived from thoracic and lumbar branches. There is considerable overlap

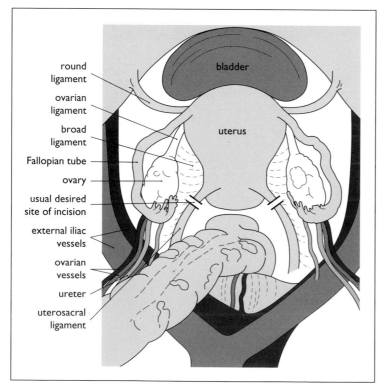

Figure 1.16 Awareness of the nerve supply in relation to the pelvic organs is important during surgery, for example, transection of the uterosacral ligaments to treat midline pelvic pain

and transversus abdominis muscles. Subsequently, these nerves pierce the rectus sheath to supply the rectus muscle (as well as internal and external obliques and transversus abdominis) and the overlying skin. The twelfth thoracic nerve often joins with the first lumbar nerve (see Figure 1.14) to form the iliohypogastric and ilioinguinal nerves, which follow paths similar to those of the lower thoracic nerves.

The lumbosacral plexus represents the neural supply from the lumbar, sacral and coccygeal portions of the pelvis. In addition, to supply the lower limbs, the plexus innervates the perineal, pudendal and coccygeal plexuses (see Figure 1.14). Knowledge of this nerve supply is important to the gynecological surgeon who attempts to treat midline pelvic pain by transection of the uterosacral ligaments, which contain afferent nerves from the uterus, or by presacral neurectomy, which involves interruption and excision of a segment of the neuroplexuses (Figure 1.16).

2 Instrumentation

Laparoscopes

Laparoscopes used during laparoscopy are of two types: a direct viewing or diagnostic laparoscope; and an operating laparoscope, which contains a central channel for passage of instruments or a laser beam (Figure 2.1). The diagnostic laparoscope (Figure 2.2) usually has a central lens surrounded circumferentially by light bundles, which provide illumination. In comparison to laparoscopes of equivalent diameter, better

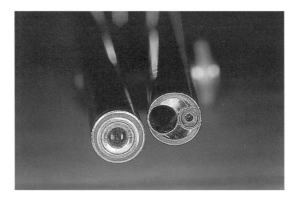

Figure 2.1 Direct viewing or diagnostic laparoscope (left) and an operating laparoscope (right) seen end-on to show the central channel

visualization is generally achieved with the diagnostic scope (because the lens diameter is larger). In an operating scope, the lens diameter is smaller to allow sufficient room for the operating channel; the light bundles are usually situated lateral to the lens.

Each type of laparoscope has an appendix near the eyepiece for attachment of the light cord. These attachments often vary according to the manufacturer; thus, it is important that the cord and laparoscope be a matched pair or that adapters be used.

Unlike a diagnostic laparoscope, which has an eyepiece at one end, operating laparoscopes have an eyepiece that is offset at either 45° or 90° (Figure 2.3). A 90° offset is further compensated by a second 90° attachment so that viewing is parallel to the barrel. Although there is no specific advantage or disadvantage between these two configurations of operating laparoscopes, each produces a slightly different orientation so that interchanging them may be difficult. Because of the parallel view of the 90°–90° offset, practitioners experienced in direct visualization through a diagnostic laparoscope may find this type more user-friendly.

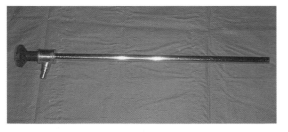

Figure 2.2 Diagnostic laparoscope

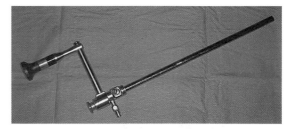

Figure 2.3 Operating laparoscope

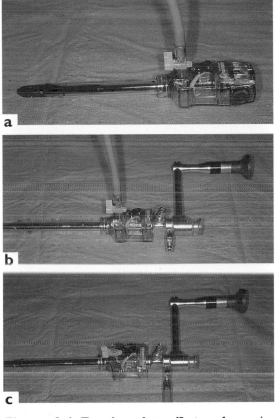

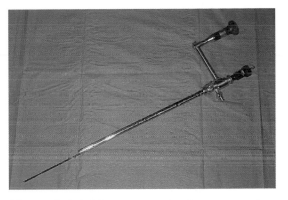

Figure 2.6 A 10-mm operating laparoscope has an additional port for other instruments

Figure 2.4 Transfer of insufflation from the laparoscopic trocar sleeve (**a** and **b**) to the laparoscope (**c**)

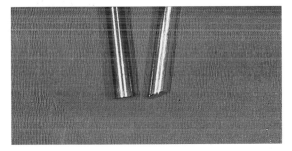

Figure 2.5 Scopes with 0° (left) and 30° (right) viewing angles

Operating laparoscopes usually have an additional appendage, an attachment for gas insufflation. It is important to use this port when using a carbon dioxide (CO_2) laser through the operating channel of the laparoscope (Figure 2.4). Gas entering the laparoscope and traversing the operating channel before exiting into the abdominal cavity minimizes entry of abdominal cavity moisture or smoke into the operating channel. Accumulation of smoke particles or moisture on the CO_2 laser lens may cause loss of the aiming beam (through absorption by moisture collected on the lens) and the deposition of carbon particles on the lens may limit the transmission of laser energy; thus, it is important to insufflate through such a port if one is available. If the intra-abdominal pressure becomes elevated, this is recognized by most insufflators with subsequent cessation of gas flow. However, raised intra-abdominal pressures can be minimized by use of insufflating gas recirculators or slight intermittent evacuations of the pneumoperitoneum to allow continuous gas inflow.

Laparoscopy may vary according to the viewing angle and diameter of the scope. Viewing angles may be 0° (end-on visualization) or 30° (Figure 2.5) and the field of view is usually 90° from these axes. The 0° angle is much more commonly used in gynecological laparoscopy. The diameter of the laparoscope is usually 5, 7 or 10 mm, with the 5- and 7-mm scopes generally used for viewing only; these do not contain operating channels. The 10-mm laparoscope (and formerly the 12 mm scope) includes space for the operat-

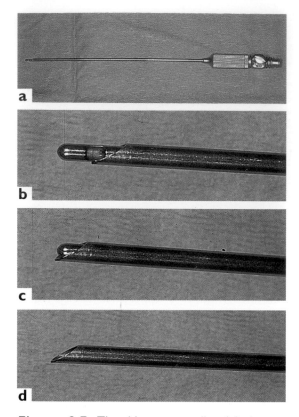

Figure 2.7 The Veress needle (**a**) has a retractable rounded sheath (**b**) which retracts (**c**) to expose a needle-like point (**d**)

ing channel, which is advantageous because it provides a portal for placement of an instrument without having to make an additional incision (Figure 2.6). However, use of these larger laparoscopes requires a larger incision in the skin and abdominal wall.

In gynecological surgery, the laparoscope is usually inserted through the umbilical incision, although other sites may be used. A narrower laparoscope (often 5 mm) can be placed through a lower abdominal or suprapubic site to allow visualization of the peritoneum where it is punctured by the umbilical instrument. Such an evaluation allows assessment of whether structures adherent to the peritoneum in the region of the umbilicus have been injured. Alternatively, these lower sites may be used to allow

tissue removal through the larger umbilical trocar sleeve or abdominal puncture site.

When using a CO_2 laser through the operating channel of an operating laparoscope, the surgeon must be aware of the presence of a blind spot. As viewing is through the lens system, bowel or other structures may obstruct the laser beam, but not lie within the field of view. In such a situation, the aiming beam of the laser (which passes parallel to the invisible CO_2 beam through the operating channel) would also not be visible. Thus, such a complication can be minimized by never firing the laser unless the aiming beam is fully visualized.

Use of monopolar electrosurgical energy through the operating channel of the laparoscope may be associated with electrosurgical injuries due to direct or capacitance coupling (see Chapter 3).

Veress needle

The Veress[*] needle (Figure 2.7 a) is a narrow instrument for insufflation of the abdominal cavity prior to placement of the laparoscopic trocar sleeve. The needle is grasped at its distal end and initially appears to have a rounded proximal end (Figure 2.7 b). However, as the proximal end is inserted into the abdominal wall, the rounded leading

---

*In an example of one of life's more unfortunate ironies, Dr János Veress, the inventor of this instrument, had the misfortune to have his name misspelled for posterity by the manufacturers of this instrument. As a consequence, Dr Veress' invention is often referred to as the 'Verres needle'. However, the correct spelling of the inventor's name can be ascertained from his original article (Veress J. Neues Instrument zur Ausführung von Brust - oder Bauchpunktionen und Pneumothoraxbehandlung. *Deutsche Med Wochenschr* 1938;64:1480–1), brought to my attention by Professor Kurt Semm of Kiel, Germany

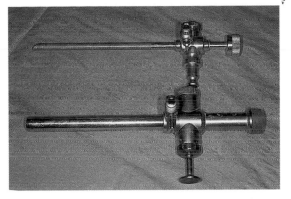

Figure 2.8 Reusable 5-mm (upper) and 10-mm (lower) trocar sleeves

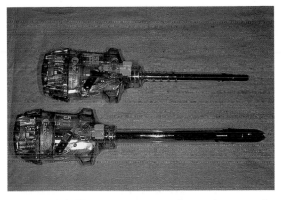

Figure 2.9 The most commonly used trocars in gynecology are 5 mm (upper) and 10 mm (lower) in diameter

edge retracts (Figure 2.7 c) to expose a needle-like point (Figure 2.7 d) which is readily able to traverse the abdominal wall to allow entry into the abdominal cavity. Immediately upon entry into the abdominal cavity, where there is no longer any abdominal wall tissue to cause its retraction, the rounded tip springs back to its original position to minimize exposure of the contents of the abdominal cavity to the sharp needle-like tip.

If the omentum, bowel or another structure is adherent to the anterior abdominal wall peritoneum at the site of puncture, the rounded tip of the Veress needle may not spring back to its original position until these attached tissues are also traversed. Thus, it is possible to cause injury to underlying tissues. Damage to non-attached underlying structures may also occur with a Veress needle either due to blunt trauma, or blunt puncture of intra-abdominal or retroperitoneal structures. Furthermore, if the rounded tip fails to spring forward (either due to instrument malfunction or inappropriate grasping of the instrument), sharp injuries may occur to these structures in the form of small puncture wounds or larger lacerations (due to manipulation once puncture has occurred). Veress needles are available in two lengths, one of which is used for the

vast majority of procedures and the other of which is of slightly longer length for use in overweight patients.

For discussions of how to assess whether the Veress needle tip is truly in the abdominal cavity, open and closed laparoscopy without the use of a Veress needle, and the method and location of placement of the Veress needle, see Chapter 5. (It should be appreciated that the extra length of the longer Veress needle potentially reduces the margin of safety if the needle is angled towards vital structures.)

Trocars and trocar sleeves

Trocar sleeves are the ports which traverse the anterior abdominal wall through which the laparoscope and other instruments are placed (Figure 2.8). Trocar sleeves are fitted with a trocar (or trocar tip) which fits snugly within it. The trocar has a sharpened tip which generally has an either pyramidal, or conical configuration. Some practitioners believe that the pyramid-shaped tip cuts through the fascia and other layers of the abdominal wall rather than tearing or pushing them aside. Thus, the conical tips are thought to be less traumatic and result in better tissue handling. However, to the

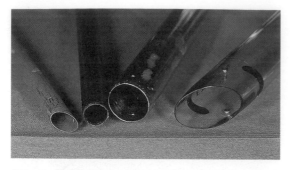

Figure 2.10 Trocar sleeves come in a range of different sizes

present author's knowledge, this purported advantage has not been demonstrated.

Trocar sleeves and their associated trocars come in several lengths and diameters. The most common diameters are 5 and 10 mm (Figure 2.9), although other diameters are available for other instruments, including some that are 3, 7, 12, 15 and 30 mm (Figure 2.10). The latter two diameters are less commonly used in gynecology. The 10-mm trocar and sleeve are available in both the standard and longer lengths (for use in overweight patients) whereas the 5-mm trocar sleeve has both standard and shortened lengths (used by some surgeons to facilitate therapeutic procedures by minimizing the length of trocar that protrudes either into the abdominal cavity or extends above the abdominal wall). Use of the standard 5-mm sleeve may result in difficulty in visualizing the instrument tip, bumping of one 5-mm trocar sleeve into another, difficulty in visualizing the pelvis, or difficulty in performing procedures in close proximity to the anterior abdominal wall.

The shorter sleeve may allow greater mobility of the trocar which may, however, make instrument exchange more difficult. Furthermore, the use of shortened 5-mm second-puncture probes may not be possible in heavier subjects because they are too short. In addition, they may frequently retract into the abdominal wall or may come away from the abdominal wall altogether, particularly during withdrawal of an instrument. For this reason, many shortened trocars (as well as some longer ones) are now manufactured with balloons, washers or other devices to allow fixation onto both the skin and peritoneal surfaces (atraumatically).

Trocar sleeves can be made of conductive materials such as metals and nonconductive materials such as most plastics. The composition of the trocar sleeve may be an important issue in some situations, for example, when there is reflection of a laser beam off the sleeve or coupling (either direct or capacitance) of electrosurgical energy (see Chapter 3 for further discussion of this topic).

Although the issue of reusable *versus* disposable instrumentation is addressed later, an attribute of many disposables that is not available on reusables is a safety shield. However, 'hybrids' are now becoming available that consist of a disposable trocar with a reusable sleeve and some of these have safety shields. The safety shield is designed to retract while the sleeve / trocar combination traverses the abdominal wall and to spring forward immediately upon entry into the abdominal cavity in much the same way that the rounded tip of the Veress needle covers the sharpened tip. Although this is theoretically advantageous, the present author is unaware of any studies which definitively demonstrate that a safety shield indeed increases safety on trocar insertion and minimizes the risk of bowel injury. (This is particularly important during placement of the first trocar sleeve in a closed procedure; subsequent trocar sleeves can be placed under direct vision as described in Chapter 5 in a discussion of closed *versus* open laparoscopy.)

Probably the most common circumstances resulting in bowel (or omental) injury during trocar placement is when these structures are directly adherent to the anterior abdominal wall peritoneum. In such situations, the safety shield is not deployed until free space is encountered and, thus, there remains the possibility of bowel (or omental) damage.

An additional attribute of the disposable (or hybrid) trocars proposed by some is that they are sharper than the usual reusable trocars. It has been demonstrated in animal studies that this results in the need to use less force to place the trocar into the abdominal cavity, which may be of particular advantage to surgeons who, because of the small size of their hands, may have difficulty in firmly grasping the trocar and sleeve or in those who have less upper body strength. However, the conclusion that the use of less force equates to less injury to underlying structures remains to be demonstrated.

Other injuries associated with trocar insertion have been anecdotally described and include blunt trauma to the bowel and mesentery as well as sharp and blunt injuries to retroperitoneal structures, including the large vessels of the pelvis and abdomen.

Blunt probes

Blunt probes are usually 5 mm in diameter and can be placed either through second-puncture trocar sleeves or down the operating channel of the laparoscope (Figure 2.11). Often, these probes have demarcations at 1-cm intervals to allow better estimation of distances and size (which may be distorted due to the viewing angle as well as the apparent magnification / demagnification of the video monitor). Blunt probes are used for atraumatic manipulation of intra-abdominal structures to improve visualization and also to retract tissue during therapeutic procedures. Hollow 'blunt probes' can be used for irrigation and / or evacuation of liquids

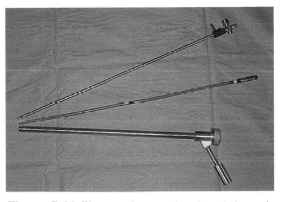

Figure 2.11 Blunt probes can be placed through a trocar sleeve or down the operating channel of a laparoscope

(such as irrigation fluid and blood) and smoke. In these circumstances, it is helpful to have additional openings on the lateral sides of the instrument to minimize the chances that abdominal structures which are sucked up will obstruct the sole aperture. The surgeon should be aware that some of the hollow probes available have sharp edges which can cut peritoneum or intra-abdominal organs during manipulation.

Scissors

Of all the instruments commonly used in endoscopic surgical procedures, scissors can be the most difficult to maintain properly. Many scissors, particularly reusable pairs, do not cut well. Thus, if only one disposable instrument were allowed for each patient, it is likely to be a pair of scissors. Hybrid scissors, with a reusable shaft but disposable blades, are also now available.

There are scissors made to fit through the operating channel of the laparoscope as well as through second-puncture trocar sleeves that are 3, 5 and 10 mm in diameter. Within these sizes, a variety of different types of scissors are available, for example, with curved or hooked tips, straight or curved blades, or flat or serrated edges

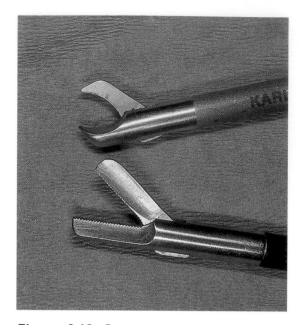

Figure 2.12 Operative scissors come with different types of blades

(Figure 2.12). The choice of which scissors to use from among these varieties is a matter of personal preference. Some believe curved blades may assist the surgeon in depth perception and may be useful in dissection. However, if the blade tips are hooked and do not cover each other when closed, the use of such scissors 'closed' for blunt dissection may result in an increased likelihood of tears or lacerations.

Scissors are configured in a number of ways. In one configuration, one blade remains fixed while the other rises to approximately 90°. In another, both blades open to equivalent degrees. Choice among these configurations again depends on physician preferences.

An additional feature available on some scissors is a shaft that is able to rotate 360° to allow manipulation of the blades to facilitate the approach to the tissue to be cut. The shaft rotation allows the surgeon to maintain the most comfortable hand position throughout the procedure. Many scissors

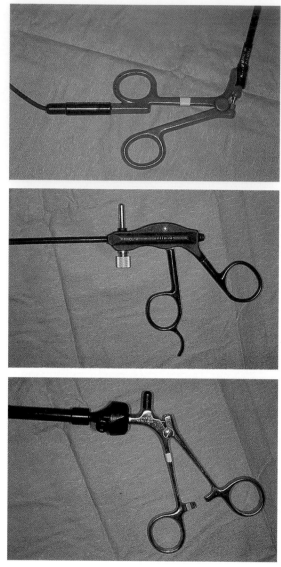

Figure 2.13 Operative laparoscopic instruments have a variety of grips and handles

are also equipped with features allowing their electrosurgical use to coagulate and cut tissue.

Handle grips

Scissors, graspers and other instruments have a variety of different types of handles (Figure 2.13). Some handles are equipped to

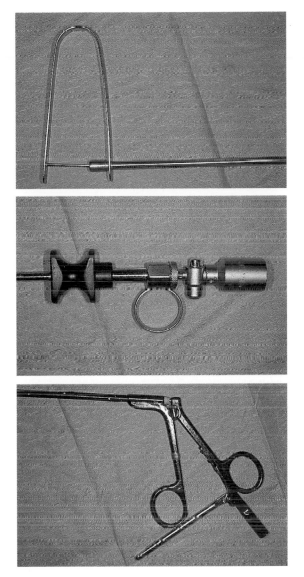

Figure 2.13 continued

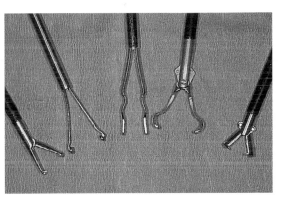

Figure 2.14 Graspers are available with a wide variety of different blade configurations

Graspers

Graspers are used to assist in tissue manipulation and retraction to allow the diagnostic evaluation and therapeutic treatment of structures in the pelvis. Although a wide variety of grasping blades are available (Figure 2.14), they generally fall into two categories. The first includes atraumatic graspers, which are usually relatively smooth and fine to minimize tissue injury. The second category includes toothed instruments, which grasp much more securely, but result in tissue damage and are therefore usually reserved for grasping tissues that are to be excised.

Tissue morcellators

Therapeutic endoscopic surgical procedures may be hindered by difficulty in removing excised tissue from the abdominal cavity. A morcellator (Figure 2.15) is an instrument which 'bites' the tissue up, thereby allowing its partial piecemeal removal. The goal is to remove sufficient amounts of tissue so as to allow the remainder to be removed through the trocar sleeve.

It is likely that morcellators are not commonly used for a variety of reasons.

allow the instrument to self-retract to maintain tension on the tissue. Such a variety has developed as a result of the individual preferences of surgeons and of the manufacturers' attempts to create comfortable, ergonomically advantageous, instruments. Again, the choice depends on physician preferences.

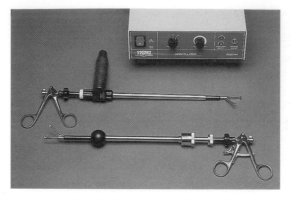

Figure 2.15 A tissue morcellator for tissue removal (courtesy of J. Deprest)

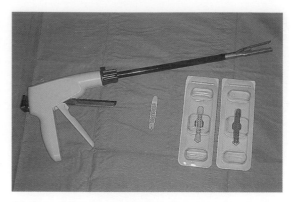

Figure 2.16 Laparoscopic linear cutter incises tissue while simultaneously placing rows of staples along each side of the incision

They require a large (10–12 mm) port and, thus, the use of a large second-puncture trocar sleeve. Alternatively, the morcellator is placed through the umbilical port (with viewing through a narrow laparoscope placed at a second puncture site). These instruments tend to be expensive and manual morcellation can be very time-consuming as well as tiring for the muscles of the forearms.

Automated morcellator systems have been evaluated, and are much more time-efficient and non-fatiguing. However, a major concern is that their use may be associated with a risk of damage (morcellation) to tissues not intended for removal. Such risk may be minimized if automated morcellation is conducted within a specimen bag, which would also minimize the risk of tissue falling back into the abdominal cavity and not being removed, with undesirable sequelae. In patients with an ectopic pregnancy, for example, failure to remove all of the tissue may lead to adherence of products of conception to intra-abdominal surfaces (such as peritoneum and endometrium) with subsequent establishment of a chronic ectopic pregnancy. Cases of ovarian cysts are another example where any excised tissue remaining within the abdominal cavity is undesirable. Alternative methods of tissue removal are discussed in Chapter 5.

Clip appliers

Clip appliers are either single- or multiple-fire, and are used to achieve hemostasis as well as to approximate tissue edges and to apply exogenous materials (such as the grafts used in hernia repairs). Clips are available in both absorbable materials (which are often able to completely surround the pedicle and require a locking mechanism) and permanent materials. Both types of clip may be associated with postoperative adhesion development, which is probably at least partly due to clip-induced tissue ischemia.

Linear cutters

Laparoscopic linear cutters (Figure 2.16) are used to staple and cut tissue pedicles. The instrument is usually able to place six parallel rows of staples simultaneously, which is followed immediately by a blade that divides the tissue between the third and fourth rows, leaving three rows on either side of the cut for hemostasis. Linear cutters are often able to use multiple cartridges with each applicator; each cartridge is used only once. The permitted thickness of pedicle that can be cut varies with the model of linear cutter used as well as the type of cartridge; some cartridges are specifically for vascular use. It is often helpful to partially dissect the pedicle to be stapled to allow closer approximation of the staples to vascularized structures.

Uterine manipulators

A wide variety of instruments is available for uterine manipulation, and there appears to be a wide range of variation among surgeons in their choice of uterine manipulators; some prefer to use instruments that others may find less useful.

The first decision to be made before choosing the best uterine manipulator for the job is whether chromotubation is to be performed. If so, the manipulator must have a channel for transit of dye. An alternative approach is to use one manipulator for chromotubation and another for the remainder of the procedure. The disadvantage, however, is the interruption of the operation to change manipulators and the time taken to replace the speculum for identification of the uterine cervical canal. In addition, there may be inadvertent vaginal contamination. Although none of these problems are major, switching uterine manipulators is usually unnecessary with careful initial instrument selection.

A reusable Cohen cannula is usually acceptable for uterine manipulation with chromotubation (Figure 2.17). Occasionally, the Cohen cannula has both a permanent 'acorn' as well as one that is removable. Placement of the cannula is carried out during direct cervical manipulation and is usually accomplished by placing a speculum with only one lateral side into the vagina after surgical preparation. The cervix is grasped at the anterior lip with a single-tooth tenaculum (see Figure 2.17), ensuring

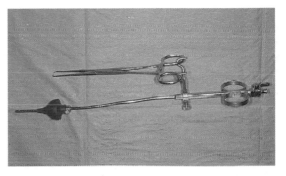

Figure 2.17 Cohen cannula attached to a tenaculum

that a large amount of tissue is grasped to minimize the likelihood of cervical tearing during uterine manipulation while taking care to avoid distortion of the cervical canal. The cannula is then positioned with the bent tip pointing towards the bladder in cases where the uterus is anteverted, or towards the bowel where the uterus is retroverted. The spring bar of the cannula is then positioned over the tenaculum (see Figure 2.17). To minimize the possibility of disengagement of the cannula from the tenaculum during procedures which are expected to involve more uterine manipulation than usual, sterile tape (if available) may be placed around the handles of these instruments to maintain their position and orientation.

Alternatives to the Cohen cannula for cervical manipulation include a variety of disposable instruments. Some of these have a balloon attached to the distal tip which can be distended once it has passed through the endocervical canal, thereby rendering a tenaculum unnecessary and reducing the egress of dye from the endocervical canal. There are at least three different varieties of such catheters: one is a rigid or semirigid rod which may also be able to accommodate weights on the handle to allow passive anteversion of the uterus; another variation is spring-loaded with a flat plate for positioning adjacent to the ectocervix; and a third

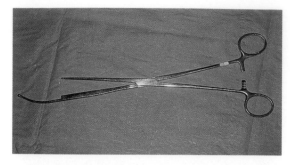

Figure 2.18 Hulka tenaculum for uterine manipulation

type has a second balloon which is positioned at the ectocervix.

With the Cohen cannula, cervical leakage of dye can be minimized by simultaneously placing traction on the tenaculum while pushing on the cannula, thereby causing occlusion at the level of the external cervical os. With the balloon-type catheters, leakage can be minimized by pulling the catheter backwards to allow the balloon to occlude at the level of the internal cervical os.

When chromotubation is not necessary, uterine manipulation can be performed with any of a range of available instruments. The Hulka tenaculum (Figure 2.18) is used by placing the long, relatively straight, blade into the cervical os while the blade at the tip grasps the cervix securely.

When using the cervical manipulators described so far, the parts of the uterus that are grasped are in the proximity of the cervix and lower uterine segment. However, at times, it may be necessary to manipulate the fundus of the uterus. One method to accomplish this is to place a tenaculum on the anterior lip of the cervix and to attach the tenaculum securely with tape to a blunt curette inserted through the cervical canal to approximately 1 cm from the apex of the uterine fundus. To minimize the likelihood of perforation with this approach, it may be helpful to use as large a (blunt) curette as will pass through the cervical canal and to back away from the apex of the fundus by 1 cm. Such an approach facilitates uterine positioning and movement by not only manipulating the cervix, but also the entire fundus.

3 Electrosurgery and laser physics: Clinical applications

Although an understanding of the physics of electrosurgical and laser equipment may appear to be superfluous to the needs of the surgeon, such knowledge will, in fact, greatly facilitate the performance of surgical procedures. At present, the goal of electrosurgical or laser energy is ultimately to cause tissue injury by the use of heat. When a high power density is achieved, the tissue at the center of the area of energy impact is vaporized (Figure 3.1). Surrounding this zone of thermal degeneration is a zone of thermal injury that is insufficient to cause total destruction; that tissue will survive, albeit with possible irreversible alterations. Finally, surrounding the zone of injury is a zone of tissue which remains undamaged by the energy source. The size of each of these zones varies according to the energy source used (based on the particular properties of the given modality) and the duration of time that the energy is applied to the tissue. Regardless of the modality, the longer the duration of energy application, the greater the size of each zone of tissue injury.

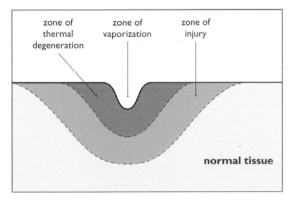

Figure 3.1 Zones of tissue injury

Electrosurgery

Electrosurgery at laparoscopy can be carried out with the use of bipolar or unipolar instrumentation (Figure 3.2). In bipolar

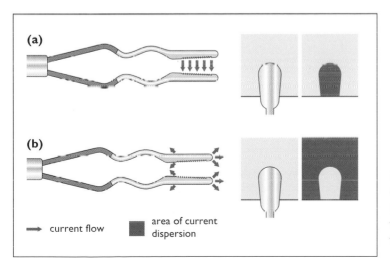

Figure 3.2 Area of current dispersion with bipolar (**a**) instrumentation is minimal compared with unipolar (**b**) instrumentation for electrosurgery

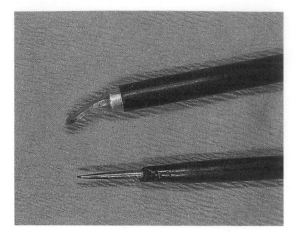

Figure 3.3 Unipolar electrosurgical instruments

instruments, the current flows from one 'jaw' to the other and, thus, the amount of tissue traversed by the energy is minimal (although some current may flow beyond the jaws). Although tissue vaporization is minimal because the power density is relatively low, zones of thermal destruction and injury may spread from the site of instrument use. Lateral extension of damage is a particular concern with more prolonged energy application because of the resultant tissue desiccation as resistance to the flow of current increases through the grasped tissue.

The most usual laparoscopic applications of bipolar electrosurgery are in tubal ligation and in the creation / establishment of hemostasis. Vascular pedicles and adhesions can be grasped and coagulated to establish hemostasis prophylactically on both sides of the site to be incised. However, as the diameter of the vessel or thickness of the pedicle / adhesion increases, the energy per unit of time imparted to tissue decreases, resulting in a greater likelihood of inadequate coaptation.

Unipolar electrosurgery employs the passage of current from the surgical instrument (Figure 3.3) to the target tissue through the pathway(s) of least resistance in the body to a return plate (the grounding pad). The

grounding pad should be placed over fleshy tissue (such as the buttock) and not at sites where bone is close to the surface (such as on the shin) or with previous surgical scars (which may have an increased resistance to current flow). The relatively large area of the grounding pad is important as it provides a greater area over which current may return from the patient to the electrosurgical generator, thereby keeping the power density low and minimizing the risk of a grounding pad-site injury.

Three formulas are important when considering the effects of electrosurgical energy on tissue: voltage = current / resistance; wattage = current × voltage; and energy imparted to tissue = wattage × time. To help in understanding these concepts, it may be helpful to imagine a water tower wherein the height of the tower represents voltage, the water in the tower represents current, and the diameter of the pipe leading from the top of the tower to the ground represents resistance. As the pipe becomes narrower, resistance to the current flow increases (or the tissue becomes desiccated) and the flow of water (current) tends to be reduced. However, this potential reduction in flow could be eliminated through compensation by increasing the height of the tower (increasing the voltage). Furthermore, if the spigot on the pipe is open only intermittently, the flow of water (current) is also intermittent and the effect on the ground (tissue) is reduced. However, this reduced effect on tissue is lost if the height of the tower (voltage) is increased. Thus, the total effect of the water (current) is the product of the height (voltage) times the period of time that the water (current) flows.

These principles can be applied to surgical procedures employing electrosurgery. The cutting current produced by an electrosurgical generator is a continuous-wave energy form of relatively low voltage.

	Name	Color	Wavelength (nm)
	Excimers	ultraviolet	200–400
	Argon	blue	488
		green	515
	532 YAG	green	532
	Krypton	green	531
		yellow	568
VISIBLE	Dye laser	yellow/green	577
		red	630
	Helium neon	red	630
	Gold vapor	red	630
	Krypton	red	647
	Ruby	deep red	694
	Nd:YAG	infrared	1064
		infrared	1318
	CO_2	infrared	10600

Figure 3.4 Positions of the currently used lasers according to wavelength in the electromagnetic spectrum

Because the voltage is low, the depth of destruction when used in a non-contact cutting mode is relatively superficial with relatively narrow zones of thermal destruction and injury. However, this benefit is offset by the fact that these cutting currents have little coagulative ability. Greater coagulative effect can be achieved by reducing the duration of current flow while increasing the voltage. The increased voltage will result in greater depth of tissue penetration with correspondingly wider zones of thermal destruction and injury. The greatest coagulative effect is achieved by tissue desiccation when the electrosurgical instrument is used in a contact mode.

Lasers

The most commonly used lasers in gynecology are the carbon dioxide (CO_2), argon, potassium titanyl–phosphate (KTP–532) and neodymium : yttrium–aluminum–garnet (Nd : YAG) lasers. Each uses a different wavelength in the electromagnetic spectrum

(Figure 3.4). Only the wavelengths used by the argon and KTP–532 lasers lie within the visible part of the spectrum. The CO_2 laser uses a helium-neon (HeNe) aiming beam to indicate where the CO_2 laser will impact upon tissue. Each of these lasers has its own properties, although the actions of the argon and KTP–532 laser are similar. Of these lasers, it is perhaps the CO_2 laser which has seen the most widespread use in gynecology.

CO_2 laser energy is usually transmitted as a beam and, although CO_2 fiber lasers have been investigated, they are generally not used routinely in clinical practice. The CO_2 laser beam is transmitted from its source to the focusing lens attached to the laparoscope through an articulated arm. There are precisely positioned mirrors at each 'joint' along the arm to transmit the focused beam from one segment to the next. Finally, the beam is transmitted through the 'knuckles' (a series of short segments which reflect the beam) to allow easy positioning of the laparoscope for use. The far end of the knuckles is attached to the lens through a

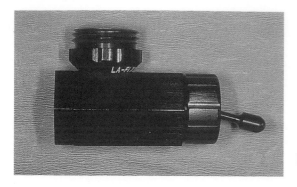

Figure 3.5 A laser coupler

coupler (Figure 3.5) either directly (if the laser arm and knuckles can be perfectly aligned) or indirectly, which allows partial manipulation of the beam. (If a perfect alignment is not possible, the coupler is then attached to the laparoscope.)

Prior to the use of the CO_2 laser in a surgical procedure, the laser should be test-fired to ensure that it is functioning correctly and that the beam is adequately aligned. The latter should be performed with the laparoscope attached because it is possible for alignment to be adequate for an open or perineal procedure with a hand-held attachment (with a short focal length), but inadequate for laparoscopic use (which requires a longer focal length; Figure 3.6). Furthermore, at this time, it should also be confirmed that the laser beam will indeed strike the same site as the aiming beam (by testing on a wet tongue blade). When these two sites do not coincide, this malalignment must be corrected before proceeding.

The CO_2 gas is introduced into the pelvis during laparoscopy either through the operating channel of the laparoscope or through a second-puncture probe; the former is more commonly used. The focal point of the CO_2 laser (the point at which the beam is most focused, thereby providing the greatest incising capability) is approximately 25 mm from the tip of the laparoscope (Figure 3.7, upper). However, because the focal length of the laser (the distance from the focusing

mirror to the focal point) is relatively long when used laparoscopically, divergence of the beam beyond the focal point is delayed (Figure 3.7, lower). As a consequence, there is a high incising capability that persists well beyond the focal point. If this is not appreciated and backstops are not appropriately positioned, then distant damage may occur. Thus, without the appropriate precautionary measures applied during lysis of adhesions of the omentum on the anterior abdominal wall, it is possible to injure the sigmoid colon deep in the pelvis.

As the effect of the CO_2 laser on tissues is relatively superficial, resulting in tissue vaporization, it is usually used for making incisions rather than for coagulation (despite a limited coagulative capability). Modulation of tissue effect can be achieved by altering the power density (energy imparted to tissue), which is influenced by the wattage (setting on the machine), spot size (distance from the focal point), and alignment of the articulating arm, knuckles and lens. Common uses of the CO_2 laser include lysis of adhesions, vaporization of endometrial implants and endometriomas, and incisions into the Fallopian tube and peritoneum.

In contrast to the CO_2 laser, the argon, KTP–532 and Nd:YAG lasers usually have their energy transmitted along fibers. The maximum power density of these fiber lasers is found at the tip of the fiber and diminishes markedly as the distance from

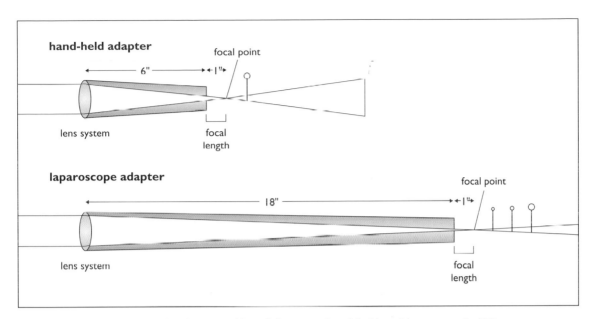

Figure 3.6 Differences in focal size and length between hand-held and laparoscopic CO_2 lasers

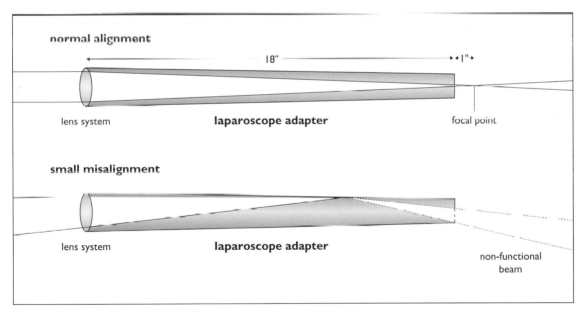

Figure 3.7 When the laser beam is properly aligned, the spot size is small at the focal point. This is not the case when the beam is misaligned

the tip increases (according to the formula: power density = wattage / $\pi 2r^2$, where r is the radius of the spot. Thus, distant structures (those lying many centimeters away from the fiber tip) are less likely to be injured with a fiber laser than with a CO_2 laser. However, because the effect of the energy from these lasers is not entirely superficial, there may be significant injury to deeper tissues lying immediately adjacent to the site of apparent tissue effect; such unintended tissue effects may not be fully appreciated at the time of surgery. The Nd:YAG laser (without the use of sculptured or sapphire tips) has a primarily coagulative effect and, thus, is mostly used in gynecology for endometrial ablation and, in general surgery, for liver resection. The use of various tips can modify the energy of the Nd:YAG laser to have a more incising, and less coagulative, effect on tissue. The argon and KTP–532 lasers have both incising and coagulative properties. Laparoscopic uses of the fiber lasers include treatment of endometriosis and adhesiolysis.

When using lasers, appropriate protection of the surgeon's eyes must be maintained. The CO_2 laser, with its superficial tissue effect, can cause damage to the cornea of the eye, although ordinary eyeglasses offer some protection (providing that the beam does not pass into the eye through the exposed sides). In contrast, fiber lasers can irreversibly damage the retina and ordinary eyeglasses will not protect against such an effect. Special lenses which absorb the specific wavelength of each particular laser beam must be used to achieve adequate protection. A scenario for the potential exposure of a surgeon's eyes that is often overlooked is when concomitant laparoscopy and hysteroscopy are performed. If the fiber laser is being used in the uterine cavity, then both the hysteroscopist and the laparoscopist need to wear eye protection in case the laser beam perforates the uterus and becomes focused by the lenses of the laparoscope onto the laparoscopist's retina, thereby causing permanent damage to the eye.

4 Preparing for laparoscopy

The operating room setup, including patient positioning, is often an area where the surgeon has, or chooses to have, little influence. Yet, this involves issues of potentially major importance as the setup can affect the conduct, ease of performance and perhaps even the efficacy of the surgical procedure. Thus, this aspect of the operation should not be overlooked by the practitioner.

Operating room setup

The appropriate equipping of the operating room will vary according to the procedure to be performed as well as the experience of the surgeon. General suggestions are listed in Table 4.1. It is important that the surgeon be familiar with all instrumentation and equipment to be used for each patient.

There are a number of different ways to organize laparoscopic equipment in the operating room; to follow is an example of one option. A cart can be obtained which houses a video monitor, video controls, light source, electrosurgical generator and insufflator. This arrangement uses a minimum amount of floor space while positioning many of the connecting cables at the back of the cart, thereby allowing light cords, insufflating tubing and video cables to approach the operating table from the same direction. In addition, an appropriate extension cord with multiple outlets for all the equipment on the cart can run from the cart to the wall outlet (providing fewer cords to trip over on the operating theater floor).

Table 4.1 Suggested instrumentation for the laparoscopic operating room

Insufflator (high flow, at least 3 L / min)
Light source
Electrosurgical generator
Video system [including camera, cord and monitor(s)]
Endoscopic instrumentation
laparoscope
graspers
scissors
irrigating probes
cervical manipulators
?Laser

Some carts position the video monitor on a movable arm, thereby providing greater flexibility in the location of the monitor. A frequently chosen location for the monitor is at the foot of the operating table during the procedure as this provides an orientation, on viewing the monitor, that is analogous to the view the surgeon would have looking directly through a laparoscope. An alternative position for the monitor is behind the first assistant which would allow the surgeon to look directly ahead to view the monitor. With this arrangement, a second monitor is often positioned behind the primary surgeon for viewing by the first assistant.

Although the use of a video monitor has a number of potential advantages, it may be equally appropriate to perform part or all of a procedure by direct viewing through the laparoscope. However, a potential advantage of using a video monitor is that it allows all operating room personnel other than the primary surgeon (for example, the surgical assistants, scrub nurse, circulating nurse and anesthesiologist) to also view the procedure. This may facilitate performance of the procedure as it allows others to see what the surgeon is trying to accomplish and, thus, helps them to provide better assistance (for instance, in the manipulation of second-puncture probes to grasp or retract tissues, or by anticipating the subsequent steps and the instruments required) as well as to remain more attentive; surgical personnel and students can also learn from direct viewing of the operative procedure. On the other hand, use of a video system increases the required capital expenditure, provides an image which many believe is adequate, but not as clear as direct viewing and, in some cases, may make performance of a procedure more difficult. However, use of a video system for operative endoscopy is becoming increasingly widespread.

A compromise between direct viewing and video-monitor viewing is to use a beam splitter which, when placed over the eye-piece of the laparoscope, allows simultaneous direct and monitor viewing. However, because of the illumination lost to the direct viewing channel, the video monitor image is often dark. This darkness can be partly overcome by using more intense light sources (such as halogen bulbs), but generally remains an important issue particularly with panoramic imaging (with close-up images, deficient illumination is less of a problem).

It is now common to find laparoscopic insufflators that supply a maximum CO_2 gas flow rate of up to 6–15 L / min. (It is important to appreciate that laparoscopic insufflators are different from hysteroscopic CO_2 gas insufflators, which have desirable flow rates that are much lower – 0.04–0.06 L /

min or 40–60 mL / min.) Although CO_2 gas is by far the most common distending medium for establishing and maintaining a pneumoperitoneum, other gases, such as nitrous oxide, may also be used. The result may be a less acidic intraperitoneal environment (by limiting formation of carbonic acid from CO_2 and water), which may lead to less diaphragmatic irritation. However, so far, there is no sound documentation to substantiate such results nor any significant differences in clinical outcome among the various gases available.

Patient positioning

The position of the patient on the operating room table should allow the anesthesiologist to monitor the patient accurately and carefully (see Chapter 16) while permitting the surgeon to perform the indicated procedure(s) efficiently and effectively. The patient may also be positioned initially according to the procedure to be performed, or she may be placed in the operative position after the induction of general anesthesia (including the placement and securing of the endotracheal tube).

To perform a laparoscopic gynecological surgical procedure, an ideal position is to have the patient's buttocks extend slightly beyond the edge of the operating table (after the foot of the table has been lowered; Figure 4.1). This facilitates the placement of instruments on the cervix for uterine manipulation. If the buttocks do not extend slightly beyond the edge of the table, it becomes difficult to antevert the uterus fully because the instrument handles will bump into the edge of the table, particularly when the patient is in the Trendelenburg position (where there is a tendency for the patient to shift towards the head of the table).

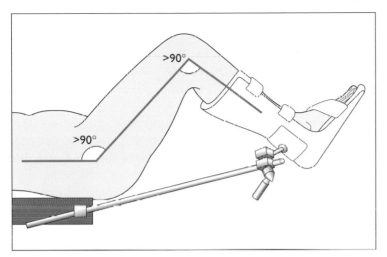

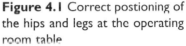

Figure 4.1 Correct postioning of the hips and legs at the operating room table

Positioning of the legs

During the induction of general anesthesia, the legs should lie straight and uncrossed. After induction of general endotracheal anesthesia and securing of the endotracheal tube, the legs can be repositioned on the stirrups after appropriate positioning of the buttocks (see above). Placing the buttocks before positioning the legs minimizes the acute angulation of the legs when repositioning the torso. The weight of the legs should rest primarily on the soles of the feet and on the ankles, thereby requiring support solely at these points or, in addition, along the calf and behind the knee. Care should be taken to ensure that there is adequate padding at weight-bearing sites to minimize the risk of injury to the skin or underlying structures, including the nerve supply and, in particular, the peroneal nerve behind the knee. The foot and ankle supports can be either straps or a heel plate.

The legs are usually positioned such that the angles between torso and thigh and between thigh and calf are both > 90° (see Figure 4.1). Some surgeons prefer to have an almost 180° angle between the torso and thigh to allow manipulation of lower-puncture probe instruments over the legs. With procedures that involve both a laparoscopic and a vaginal approach, such as a laparoscopically assisted vaginal hysterectomy (LAVH), a different position may be used initially from that used during the latter portions of the procedure.

Positioning of the arms

The arms may be placed in one of three positions during the operative procedure:

(1) At approximately 90° to the torso, extending perpendicularly from the body;

(2) Alongside the body, extending down the length of the torso; or

(3) Folded across the chest.

Choosing which of these positions to use depends upon the personal preferences of the surgeon and anesthesiologist as well as the procedure to be performed.

During therapeutic procedures and particularly if the video monitor is not to be used, it is preferable to have at least one of the patient's hands not extending perpendicularly from the body. This allows the surgeon to move along the side of the table, thereby facilitating performance of the procedure and minimizing back strain during more prolonged procedures. Placing both arms either alongside the patient's torso or across the patient's chest provides the same benefits to the surgical assistant. However, these positions tend to limit access to intravenous lines that are inserted in the hand, should any intravenous difficulties arise. Placing the hands across the chest removes them to where they do not obstruct the surgeon while remaining accessible to the anesthesiologist. However, this hand position may interfere with manipulation of either the instruments or the laparoscope and may, it has been suggested, decrease patient ventilation.

Trendelenburg position

The Trendelenburg position allows bowel and other intra-abdominal structures to shift cephalad, thereby increasing visualization of the pelvis. Usually, the greater the degree of the position, the more visualization is increased. However, this position, particularly when held at excessive degrees, may increase the weight of intra-abdominal structures on the diaphragm and limit diaphragmatic excursion, thereby impeding patient ventilation. Thus, the operating surgeon and anesthesiologist need to agree on a patient position based on characteristics such as body habitus, weight and cardiovascular status.

An additional potential problem with larger degrees of the Trendelenburg position is the shift of the patient's body towards the head of the operating table. This can be minimized by the use of shoulder braces, although there has been some concern that some braces may predispose to nerve injuries.

After sterile draping of the patient, the cart bearing the laparoscopic equipment can be positioned at the foot of the table, and the tables for the light source and video monitor as well as the insufflating gas tubing can be brought closer to the operative field. Any other equipment required for the operative procedure can then be positioned.

For patients who are to undergo combination hysteroscopy and laparoscopy, the order in which these procedures are carried out will vary according to the clinical situation. Often, hysteroscopy precedes or is performed concurrently with laparoscopy. This allows laparoscopic viewing of the serosa of the uterus during the therapeutic hysteroscopy (for a more detailed description, see Chapter 7, *A Manual of Clinical Hysteroscopy* by R.F. Valle). Laparoscopy during hysteroscopy is believed to minimize the risk of uterine perforation while allowing identification of perforation should it occur and, thus, minimizing the risk of damage to intraperitoneal structures by allowing a timely identification of injuries to bowel or other intra-abdominal structures. Nonetheless, laparoscopy is not routinely carried out during hysteroscopic procedures because of the potential morbidity associated with laparoscopy.

5 Initiating the procedure

In preparation for initiation of the surgical procedure, attention must be directed to where the incisions are to be made. Most commonly, the laparoscopic trocar is placed at or immediately below the umbilicus. This area, as well as the areas where second-puncture probes will be placed, is prepared with a surgical dressing solution to minimize bacterial content. This is accomplished with a surgical scrub followed by painting of the surface with a final solution. 'Prepping' is usually carried out by first preparing the sites where the surgical incisions will be made, which is then followed by the areas extending away from the sites of incisions, thus pushing the bacteria away from the sites where incisions are to be made. If body surfaces are dried with a sterilized towel, the towel should always be lifted by the edges for removal to avoid contamination of the prepared incisional sites. Sterilized towels should never be grabbed in the center and lifted as this method allows the edges of the towel to traverse the abdominal wall before being lifted away.

Depending on the intended locations of the second-puncture incisions, the patient's pubic hair may be trimmed prior to preparation of the abdominal wall. Although there is no evidence that this has any beneficial effect on the infection rate at the sites of incision, the subsequent skin closure is facilitated without having to cope with the entrapment of hair.

The bladder may be drained at the time of vaginal preparation. Even if a patient has been NPO (nothing by mouth) overnight, the intravenous fluid administered prior to initiation of the procedure may result in a large volume of urine in some patients. If the bladder is distended, there is an increased risk of injury to the bladder during placement of the second puncture trocars. Thus, it may be useful to drain the bladder prior to initiating the procedure. In patients in whom prolonged procedures or surgery surrounding the bladder are considered likely, a Foley catheter may be placed to allow evaluation of urinary output as well as identification of hematuria, should it occur. The catheter will also help to minimize the likelihood of bladder distention during the procedure which may interfere with the operation.

Abdominal and perineal / vaginal preparation may be carried out simultaneously by two operating room personnel, or by one person who first prepares the abdomen, then the perineum / vagina. As with the abdominal wall, the perineum / vagina is prepared with a scrubbing solution followed by a prepping solution. After preparation of the vagina, a speculum is placed to identify the cervix. The cervix is grasped usually by the anterior lip, using a single-tooth tenaculum and taking a sufficiently large amount of tissue so as to minimize the risk of tearing during uterine manipulation.

After placing the tenaculum, an instrument for chromotubation is positioned in the cervical canal, usually a Cohen cannula, although a number of alternatives are available (see Chapter 2). The Cohen cannula can be taped (using sterile tape) to the tenaculum to minimize the likelihood of their becoming separated due to their being manipulated during the surgical procedure. (Should separation occur, usually both the speculum and cannula need to be repositioned on the cervix.)

Prior to the initial skin incision, the anesthesiologist may temporarily place a nasogastric or orogastric tube to ensure that the stomach does not become distended during the process of intubation. If the stomach becomes distended with gas, there is thought to be an increased risk of perforation of the stomach during placement of either the Veress needle or the laparoscopic trocar.

Locating the initial incision

The most common location for placement of the laparoscopic trocar sleeve is at the umbilicus. The umbilical incision can be either vertical, horizontal or crescent-shaped along the inferior curvature of the umbilicus (Figure 5.1). The size of the initial incision may be just enough to allow introduction of the Veress needle or large enough to allow placement of the upper laparoscopic trocar sleeve. A large incision initially eliminates

the need to reobtain the scalpel to lengthen the initial incision. However, oozing may occur during insufflation with the Veress needle. The choice of incision is usually by surgeon preference. Whereas some surgeons always use the same incision, others prefer to vary the choice based on the appearance of the patient's umbilicus to minimize visibility of the resultant incisional scar. Placing the incision deep within the umbilicus improves later cosmetic appearances, as it will be less noticeable, although closure is then slightly more time-consuming upon completion of the procedure.

Once the skin incision has been made, the Veress needle is placed by grasping the needle at its upper portion to allow the proper function of its safety features (see Figure 2.7, Chapter 2). However, an apparently increasingly used alternative to the Veress needle is direct trocar insertion without prior establishment of a pneumoperitoneum. After the Veress needle has been placed in the incision, the abdominal wall is elevated for deeper insertion of the needle. It is usually possible to feel when the fascia and then the peritoneum have been traversed by the Veress needle.

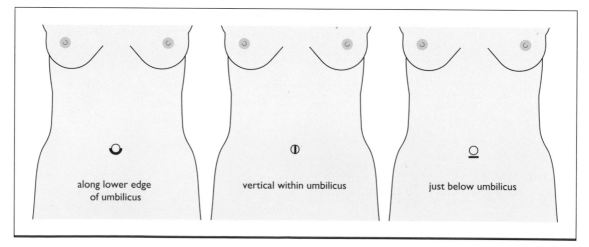

Figure 5.1 Umbilical skin incisions for laparoscopic trocar placement

Attempts should be made to ascertain the position of the tip of the needle by, for example, first injecting saline or other irrigating solution through a syringe, then attempting to draw the fluid back into the syringe. Fluid is more likely to be drawn when the tip of the needle lies preperitoneal than when in the abdominal cavity, where the fluid would be dispersed throughout the cavity. If a substantial amount of blood is obtained, then vascular injury must be considered. If a brownish foul-smelling fluid is obtained, then bowel injury must be considered. Another technique to establish needle-tip position is to place a drop of irrigating solution on the hub of the Veress needle. Then, when the abdominal wall is elevated and the needle lies free within the abdominal cavity, the clinging drop of fluid should fall freely into the cavity. A third alternative is to attach the insufflation tubing to the Veress needle before insufflation. At a rate of approximately 1 L / min, the intra-abdominal pressure should be < 10 mmHg. If the resultant pressures are higher than this, then some form of obstruction to flow should be considered either at the level of the tubing, within the Veress needle or at the tip of the needle if it lies outside the abdominal cavity or up against an intraperitoneal structure. When gas insufflation is at a rate > 1 L / min, it is possible to obtain higher intra-abdominal pressure recordings of gas flow due to the small diameter of the Veress needle. On confirmation of an intra-abdominal position of the needle tip, the rate of gas insufflation can be increased to minimize the time taken to achieve an adequate pneumoperitoneum.

It should be borne in mind that, with any of these techniques to ascertain the position of the Veress needle tip, it is possible to be misled. Even if all of the suggested options were to be used, appropriate placement of the needle is not guaranteed.

Usually, 3–4 L of CO_2 gas are required to establish an adequate pneumoperitoneum. Instead of checking the volume of gas instilled, an adequate pneumoperitoneum may be assessed by the loss of liver dullness during percussion over the liver and by noting a change in abdominal wall girth. However, these physical signs may be difficult in obese patients. When an adequate degree of pneumoperitoneum appears to be established, the Veress needle is removed, and the laparoscopic trocar and sleeve placed. During trocar placement, it is often possible to feel a snap each time that the fascia and peritoneal layers are traversed. Furthermore, with some trocars, a flow of gas from the abdominal cavity is registered when the cavity is entered (or from the preperitoneal space if insufflated with gas).

When the trocar and sleeve are in place, the trocar is removed and the laparoscope inserted through the sleeve. The surgeon initially confirms the intra-abdominal placement of the laparoscope. Inspections should then be performed beneath the laparoscope as well as circumferentially around the site of trocar placement to ascertain whether underlying structures, such as the omentum and bowel, have been injured. Evaluation is finally performed to determine whether there are any adhesions to the anterior abdominal wall. If adhesions are noted in the vicinity of the umbilicus, then the surgeon must confirm whether the trocar traversed the bowel prior to entry into the abdominal cavity. Such injury can be confirmed or ruled out by visualization either through the umbilical port or through a laparoscope at the second puncture site.

Alternative methods of primary trocar insertion

The preceding description of trocar placement covered the most common method;

however, there are alternatives. Some surgeons place the trocar directly without prior abdominal insufflation. In this case, the abdominal wall is elevated at the site where the trocar is to be placed. The trocar is then advanced through the previously made skin incision in a similar manner as with insufflation. After placement, the trocar is removed, the laparoscope positioned, the abdomen insufflated and the cavity examined to assess whether any underlying structures have been injured before proceeding with the laparoscopic procedure.

Both the traditional method of entry as well as the direct trocar insertion method involve placement of a central laparoscopic trocar sleeve without being able to visually determine whether any structures are adherent to the peritoneum at the intended site of entry. (There are, however, techniques of Veress needle placement that can be used in the attempt to assess whether adherent structures are present.)

Some surgeons advocate the use of 'open' laparoscopy, in which the primary trocar site is created by a skin incision that is dissected down sharply into the peritoneum. Although it is suggested that this technique will reduce the incidence of inadvertent injury to bowel and other underlying structures, this has never, to my knowledge, been demonstrated in well-designed clinical trials. The literature to date, in fact, does not appear to support any demonstrable benefit of 'open' *versus* 'closed' laparoscopy. Indeed, there have been anecdotal reports of dissection into bowel with the open technique and even reports of such injury going unrecognized during performance of the surgical procedure.

With the open technique, the trocar sleeve is placed as soon as the abdominal cavity is pierced. Because the incisions in the abdominal wall and peritoneum are generally larger than the diameter of the trocar sleeve, the incision must be closed round the sleeve to allow creation of a pneumoperitoneum. This is accomplished by a specially designed cannula which allows sutures to be tied at each side of the trocar. Alternatively, the fascia of the abdominal wall can be sutured on each side to prevent leakage of gas around the trocar sleeve.

Finally, a device has recently been introduced to facilitate primary trocar placement. After having made the skin incision, the device is placed in the defect. The tip of the device is open to allow viewing of the underlying tissue with the laparoscope. The surgeon slowly advances the device by cutting the tissue with a blade at the tip of the device. This blade is only exposed when a trigger is squeezed and incises only an extremely thin layer of tissue. This device thus allows the surgeon to visualize the peritoneum (and any adherent structures) before incision. It remains to be seen whether this innovation will indeed reduce the incidence of inadvertent injury to underlying structures in well-designed clinical trials.

Secondary trocar placement

After assessing the region of the umbilicus, attention should be directed to those areas of the anterior abdominal wall intended for second-puncture probes to confirm whether these areas are free of adhesions. If adhesions are noted, the surgeon may decide to choose another site for the second-puncture probes, or, alternatively, to remove the adhesions. Depending on the procedure to be undertaken, the second-puncture probes may be placed either in the midline or laterally, and at any level above the pubic symphysis.

Usually, secondary probes are placed immediately above the pubic hair line either in the midline or lateral to the midline. When placing secondary probes lateral to the midline, consideration must be given to the

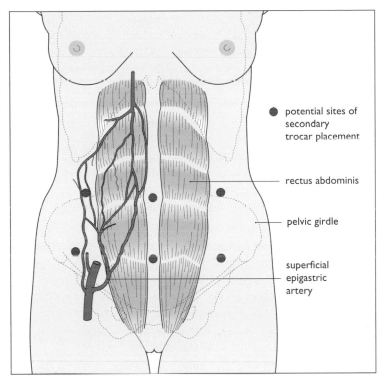

potential sites of
secondary
trocar placement

rectus abdominis

pelvic girdle

superficial
epigastric
artery

Figure 5.2 Potential locations for
secondary trocar placement

paths taken by the inferior epigastric vessels
(Figure 5.2). Whereas some practitioners
suggest that these vessels can be identified
by transillumination, others may find
difficulty in doing so. Although the superficial epigastric vessels may be identifiable
in non-obese patients, the deep inferior
epigastric vessels will remain difficult to
identify. As a rule, the inferior epigastric
vessels tend to run immediately adjacent to
the obliterated umbilical vessels. Thus, placement of a second-puncture probe at this site
needs to be carried out with caution and only
after prior attempts to visualize the vessels
laparoscopically during direct palpation of
the area.

Despite these precautions, damage to
the epigastric vessels is still possible. Several
methods have been suggested to control
bleeding of the epigastric vessels. One option
is to cut through the skin to the site of the
vessels, identify the site of bleeding and tie

off the bleeding vessels. An alternative is to
place an electrosurgical instrument or clip
through another second-puncture site to
grasp the bleeding vessel and establish
hemostasis via coagulation or clipping.
Suturing the vessels has also been suggested,
using either through-and-through sutures
from the abdominal wall (although anecdotal
evidence from patients suggests that such
sutures are extremely painful) or suturing
intra-abdominally. A final alternative is to
place a Foley catheter through the second-
puncture trocar sleeve at the site of the
bleeding vessels. The balloon is distended
with saline and pulled up to the abdominal
wall; a clamp is then placed on the catheter
at the skin surface to exert pressure on the
bleeding vessels. Some surgeons report
leaving clamps in place for as long as
approximately 24 h, although delayed passage of clots from such sites has also been
described.

6 Diagnostic evaluation of the pelvis

In the healthy, hemodynamically stable patient, evaluation of the pelvis is usually performed after placement of the initial second-puncture probe(s). In patients with pelvic pathology, evaluation may initially be limited until adhesions are lysed or other pathology is treated. When pathology does not limit evaluation, it is preferable to complete the diagnostic evaluation before initiating any indicated therapy to minimize the likelihood of any areas being overlooked.

A useful recommendation is to develop a routine to follow of the order in which the areas of the pelvis are evaluated to further ensure that no areas are missed. As an example of such a routine, after placement of the umbilical and second-puncture trocar sleeves, the uterus is retroverted to allow examination of the peritoneum of the anterior cul-de-sac for the presence of adhesions and endometriosis (Figure 6.1). Similar examinations are made of the anterior, followed by the posterior, uterine surfaces while noting uterine size and contour as well as location and size of any myomas found.

Next, after replacing the uterus to an anteverted position, the posterior cul-de-sac, uterosacral ligaments and anterior surface of the sigmoid colon are evaluated in turn for adhesions and endometriosis. Engorged vessels (suggested by some to be associated with pelvic pain in the pelvic congestion syndrome) and peritoneal pockets (thought by some to represent endometriotic implants) are also sought.

Attention is then directed to the adnexa, beginning with those on the left. The uterus is manipulated to a position contralateral to the side being investigated. The entire Fallopian tube is examined for the presence of adhesions (Figure 6.2) and endometriosis. Elevation and firmness (noted with a second-puncture probe) at the point of tubal insertion into the uterus may indicate salpingitis isthmica nodosa (SIN), a condition in which the lumen of the tube appears to have multiple small fenestrations and is associated with a reduction in fertility. To view the whole of its surface, the tube often needs manipulation. The tip of the second-puncture probe can be used to gently lift the distal end of the tube, thereby permitting the medial portion of the tube, and peritoneum lying between the tube and ovary, to be investigated. The presence of paratubal cysts, accessory fimbria, tubal fistulas, tubal abscesses and ectopic pregnancy should also be sought. The distal or infundibular part of the tube is then evaluated for the presence of a hydrosalpinx or tubal phimosis. Finally, the fimbria are macroscopically examined for evidence of intrafimbrial scarring or adhesive bands as well as to assess the appearance of the fimbria themselves for areas of, for example, tubal baldness.

Next, the ovary is evaluated in terms of size, surface characteristics (smoothness), and the presence of adhesions (see Figure 6.2), surface endometriotic implants and endometriomas, bearing in mind that it is often difficult to distinguish between a corpus luteum and an endometrioma. As

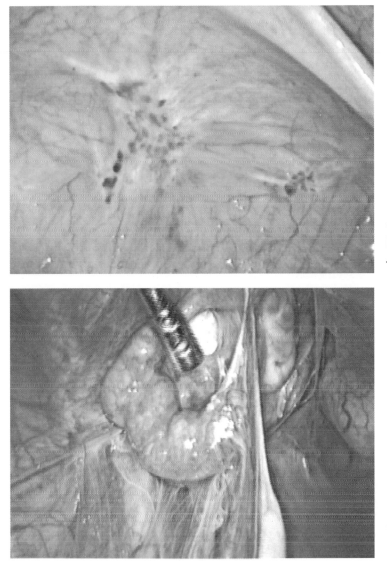

Figure 6.1 Endoscopic view of endometriotic implants on the peritoneum (courtesy of D.A. Johns)

Figure 6.2 Endoscopic view of ovarian and tubal adhesions (courtesy of D.A. Johns)

with the Fallopian tube, a full evaluation requires gentle elevation of the ovary to assess the underside of the ovary as well as the underlying ovarian fossa. This can be accomplished by use of a second-puncture probe, positioned at either the proximal or distal ovarian pole, to gently roll the ovary upwards and out of the way. It is imperative that the ovary and tube be manipulated gently as punctate inflammation and / or bleeding may occur due to rubbing of the instrument along peritoneal surfaces. Signif-

icant bleeding or tissue trauma can be induced by instruments even when they are blunt (such as irrigating probes). The remaining parts of the broad ligament and pelvic side wall are then evaluated.

After examining the left adnexa, the uterus is repositioned, using a uterine manipulator, to the left side of the pelvis to allow examination of the right adnexa, following the same system as was used on the left. In some women, the appendix lies in the vicinity of the right adnexa and should

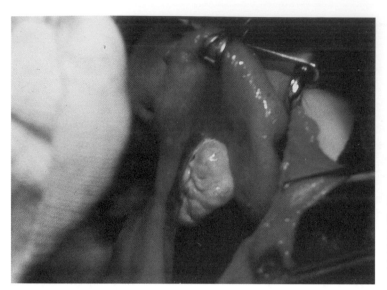

Figure 6.3 Classical 'frog's eggs' appearance of the mesosalpinx, in this case, due to chlamydial infection (courtesy of A.H. DeCherney)

also be evaluated. Thus, the diagnostic evaluation of the pelvis can be described as following an alpha-shaped pattern.

The upper abdomen can also be examined for the presence of endometriosis or adhesions. The appearance of 'violin-string' adhesions, frequently asymptomatic, from the surface of the liver to the overlying peritoneum is called the Fitz-Hugh–Curtis syndrome and is thought to be a sequela of pelvic infection. Visualization of the upper abdomen will also allow identification of the hepatoumbilical ligament, which runs from the umbilicus to the liver and represents the vestigial remnant of the left umbilical vein.

In infertility patients, chromotubation is performed through the manipulatory cannula placed in the cervical os. The chromotubating solution usually contains indigo–carmine dye as, on rare occasions, the use of methylene blue has been associated with the development of methemoglobin. Chromotubation can be performed by the circulating nurse or other non-scrubbed personnel if the external surface of the dye syringe is not kept sterile. Alternatively, if sterility has been maintained

and the syringe has not been contaminated, the surgeon or other scrubbed personnel can inject the dye.

During chromotubation, a tight cervical seal needs to be maintained (see Chapter 2) to prevent the egress of dye from the cervix with the possible result that the dye will then fail to fill and spill from the Fallopian tubes. If such failure should occur, occlusion of the cervix should be reconfirmed and injection at a higher pressure attempted. If the tubes are patent, then dye will readily be seen to fill and spill from them; if dye is seen to exit from only one tube, an attempt can be made, using a second-puncture instrument, to temporarily occlude the patent tube to determine whether the non-filling tube will then fill and spill.

Any abnormalities of the tubes may also be identified during chromotubation which were not otherwise noted previously. Examples include patients with partial distal tubal occlusion in whom dye can be seen to spill (and fimbria are noted, but the ampullary and / or infundibular portion of the tube becomes distended) during chromotubation. The failure of dye to pass freely may indicate intratubal pathology which may lead to an inability to conceive. Occasionally, a 'sausage-link' or 'frog's eggs' appearance (Figure 6.3) is identified during chromotubation in which the tubal wall appears to be extremely thin; this may indicate patients with tubal mucosal damage.

A major challenge facing endoscopic surgeons is how to remove excised tissue from the abdominal cavity. This problem arises following such procedures as salpingectomy, oophorectomy, ovarian cystectomy and myomectomy. Tissues that are small, narrow and / or malleable can be extracted through the second-puncture trocar sleeve grasped by an endoscopic instrument. If the trocar sleeves are too narrow to allow such extraction, a number of alternatives can be considered:

(1) Endoscopic instruments can be used to cut the tissue up into smaller pieces that will fit through the trocar sleeves. This can be accomplished before as well as after excision of the tissue. The disadvantage of delayed excision is specimen bleeding; however, it allows fixation of the tissue which facilitates dissection;

(2) A narrow laparoscope can be placed through a small secondary-puncture trocar, thereby allowing a grasping instrument to be placed through the larger primary umbilical trocar sleeve. Tissue can thus be removed through the umbilical port;

(3) Tissue can be morcellated using a morcellator, which can be either powered by hand or mechanically;

(4) Tissue can be removed through the vagina subsequent to a posterior colpotomy incision. This incision traverses the posterior vaginal wall and can be created either laparoscopically or vaginally. Viewed laparoscopically, the incision is made immediately inferior to the insertion of the uterosacral ligaments into the cervix; viewed vaginally, the incision is in the posterior fornix;

(5) After grasping the tissue, the trocar sleeve can be removed to allow the specimen to be 'teased' through the abdominal wall defect;

(6) A minilaparotomy incision can be made to allow tissue removal after laparoscopic excision.

Further consideration is required as to whether the tissue should be morcellated (or a cyst ruptured) to facilitate its removal as doing so increases the potential of such tissue falling into the abdominopelvic cavity. This is of particular concern in women treated laparoscopically for ectopic pregnancy by salpingostomy or salpingectomy, as trophoblast reimplantation has been described in the pelvic peritoneum and omentum.

Furthermore, if malignant tissue is morcellated and incompletely removed from the abdominal cavity, the clinical outcome is poor. To minimize the risk of retained tissue, a bag has been devised which can be placed laparoscopically through a trocar. After the specimen has been placed in the bag, it can then be removed through a trocar sleeve. Any tissue or fluid dislodged or expressed from the specimen during removal will then be retained in the bag rather than falling back into the abdominal cavity. Alternatively, tissue can be morcellated while in the bag so that no fragments are lost. This helps to ensure complete removal of the specimen.

Procedure completion

After completing the diagnostic evaluation, attention should then be directed to treatment of the pathology identified during

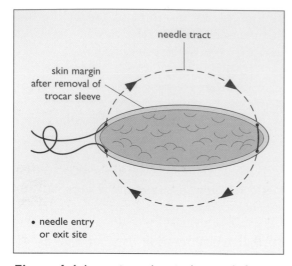

Figure 6.4 A running subcuticular stitch for use in longer incisions

examination. If no pathology is present or therapy has been completed, the procedure can then be terminated. Prior to removal of the trocar sleeves, the operative sites may be reexamined to ascertain that no active bleeding remains and no unintended (and untreated) tissue or organ damage has occurred. Frequently, irrigation is helpful as it will wash away any blood. Some surgeons leave behind a large volume of fluid in the abdominal cavity as a matter of routine whereas others will never do so. The purported advantages of leaving fluid behind are that it reduces the likelihood of postoperative adhesions and postoperative pain, the latter by minimizing retention of CO_2 gas in the abdomen and thereby decreasing diaphragmatic irritation. However, thus far, the data substantiating these claims are not convincing. Indeed, patients who are left with a large volume of fluid in the abdominal cavity are often alarmed by leakage from the trocar incision sites.

On completion of reevaluation of the pelvis, closure can proceed first by releasing the distending CO_2 gas and then by removal of the second-puncture trocar sleeve(s). The peritoneal surface surrounding the second-puncture site(s) should also be inspected for bleeding. Finally, the umbilical trocar sleeve is removed and closed with a deep 'fascial' stitch, followed by closure of all skin incisions. In general, deep stitches are not used at 5-mm trocar sites and most surgeons appear to concur with placing deep stitches at all trocar sites that are $\geq 10\,$mm to minimize the risk of incisional hernias. Skin closure may be accomplished with mattress stitches that encompass both skin and subcutaneous tissue, although some surgeons prefer to place a subcuticular stitch that does not require removal. Such a subcuticular stitch may consist of a 'running' stitch such as used for longer incisions, although one or two interrupted stitches (Figure 6.4) will also suffice.

To minimize postoperative incisional pain, some surgeons suggest infiltration of the incision site with a local anesthetic such as bupivacaine (Marcaine™). Finally, sterile strips or adhesive tapes can be applied over the incision. If skin-edge oozing is noted, a small pressure dressing can be applied. During closure of the abdominal incision, all vaginal instruments are also removed. Care should be taken when repositioning the patient to avoid injury to the extremities. In particular, if the patient's arms have lain at her sides, the fingers should be carefully guarded to avoid their being caught as the tilt of the lower end of the table is repositioned to horizontal.

7 Ectopic pregnancy

The diagnosis of ectopic pregnancy can be difficult to make. The importance of making the diagnosis, however, is emphasized by the potential dire outcome if diagnosis is made too late, as the ectopic pregnancy may rupture with resultant hemorrhage and possible death. On the other hand, if the diagnosis is made too soon, it may not be possible to identify the eccyesis on diagnostic laparoscopy. Although a detailed discussion of the diagnostic work-up of ectopic pregnancy is beyond the scope of this book, the reader should be aware that the diagnosis is based on a combination of history, physical examination, serial β-human chorionic gonadotropin (β-hCG) measurements and ultrasound scans as well as other diagnostic information. For a more complete review of the options and use of diagnostic modalities for determination of ectopic pregnancy, the reader is referred to recent publications.

When the clinical suspicion of an eccyesis is, on the basis of the diagnostic work-up, sufficiently strong and the clinician has decided to treat by surgical intervention, consideration needs to be given to the mode of entry to the abdominal cavity. For the patient who is in hemorrhagic shock, the most expedient method of abdominal entry to rapidly control bleeding should be used; for the vast majority of practitioners, this will probably be by emergency laparotomy. However, when the patient is hemodynamically stable, laparoscopy may be considered to be the optimal means for a definitive diagnosis of ectopic pregnancy and its subsequent treatment.

A tubal ectopic pregnancy often appears as a tubal bulge with a bluish hue. On occasions, the serosa of the tube may be ruptured and bleeding even though the patient is hemodynamically stable. In other patients, the tube may be bleeding from the fimbriated end. Many ectopic pregnancies, however, will have no bleeding and remain intact.

The choice of surgical procedure, either salpingostomy or salpingectomy, should be based on the patient's desire for future pregnancy, the size of the eccyesis and the extent of tubal damage. In the patient who is bleeding, evacuation of the hemoperitoneum will allow greater visualization of the tube. However, if it appears that the patient may become hemodynamically unstable, achieving vascular control should then become a priority.

There are numerous options for the endoscopic treatment of ectopic pregnancy. This chapter includes only a small selection out of many alternatives. The treatment of ectopic pregnancy via the laparoscope is frequently performed with either a two- or three-puncture technique, depending on the experience and expertise of the surgeon and on characteristics of the eccyesis itself.

The most common site for an ectopic pregnancy is in the ampullary segment of the Fallopian tube (Figure 7.1). To treat an ampullary eccyesis by salpingostomy, the tube should be grasped, using a self-retaining grasping instrument, distal to the site of the pregnancy. This is usually easily accomplished by inserting an instrument

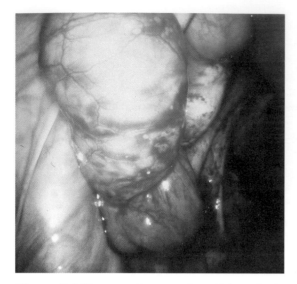

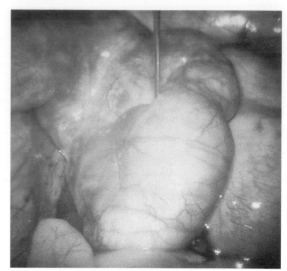

Figure 7.1 The ampullary portion of the tube is enlarged and fusiform, an appearance consistent with a tubal gestation (courtesy of V. Gomel)

Figure 7.2 The mesosalpinx adjacent to the gestational site is infiltrated with diluted vasopressin (courtesy of V. Gomel)

through a port ipsilateral to the site of the eccyesis to avoid interference with instruments inserted through other ports or with the line of vision. When tension is placed on the tube, the size of the pregnancy can be assessed and decisions made as to whether to attempt salpingostomy and whether to use synthetic vasopressin. For the practitioner who is lacking experience with laparoscopic treatment of ectopic pregnancies, the general indications for laparoscopic management include an ectopic pregnancy that is ≤3 cm in diameter, a tube free of adhesions and a hemodynamically stable patient.

If synthetic vasopressin is to be used to reduce intraoperative bleeding, the agent may be injected through either an instrument inserted via a second-puncture probe or via the operative channel of the laparoscope or via a spinal needle. Although synthetic vasopressin has not been officially approved for this indication, it is nevertheless often used in diluted form. Among the variety of concentrations used, one option is to use 1 ampoule (20 units) of synthetic vasopressin

in 100 mL of saline. This is injected into the antimesenteric border of the Fallopian tube (Figure 7.2).

If a spinal needle is used for injecting, it is important first to identify by palpation the site of the depression in the abdominal wall which indicates the location of the tube. The spinal needle is then placed at this depression at the appropriate angle to bring the needle tip within proximity of the tube. Fine adjustments can be made by moving the tube, using a grasping instrument at the distal end of the Fallopian tube. (It is important to ensure that the grasping instrument is in contact with the serosa of the tube and not the fimbria.) Some surgeons prefer to inject vasopressin into the mesosalpinx to reduce the blood supply to the tube whereas others prefer not to use synthetic vasopressin at all, maintaining that if the site of the eccyesis is going to bleed, it is preferable that it occurs during the operation while the surgeon is present than when the vasopressin wears off in the recovery room.

An incision that is approximately two-thirds the length of the eccyesis is made in the Fallopian tube (Figure 7.3). The incision can be made by any modality according to the surgeon's preference – electrosurgery, laser or scissors. There is no firm evidence that any of these modalities produces superior results compared with the others. In some patients, the products of conception begin to extrude from the incision immediately after it has been made. These products can be grasped with an appropriate instrument and removed through the laparoscopic trocar. If the tissue is not extruded on its own, an irrigating probe can be placed in the incision and the tissue irrigated to facilitate dissection. Alternatively, the grasping instrument can be inserted into the incision to retrieve the products of conception. The surgeon must take care when placing the grasping instrument in the tube as it is possible to avulse tissue that is not part of the eccyesis. Should this occur, the result is often excessive bleeding that requires electrosurgery to achieve hemostasis and significant damage to the Fallopian tube.

After all of the easily evacuable tissue has been removed, some surgeons irrigate the pregnancy bed in an attempt to free additional tissue. Others use grasping instruments within the incision to remove whatever tissue is easily detached. Overly aggressive attempts to remove tissue are to be avoided because of the possible bleeding which may be initiated. However, persistent ectopic pregnancies occur in approximately 5–10% of patients and may be the result of inadequate removal of trophoblastic tissue from the ectopic bed. Thus, thorough evacuation of the ectopic site should be attempted with minimal loss of such tissue into the abdominal cavity. The latter is particularly important because there have been several reports of trophoblastic tissue becoming implanted within the abdominal cavity on

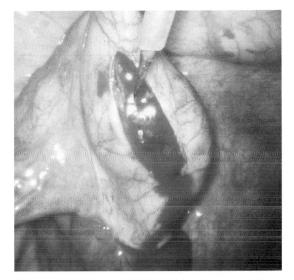

Figure 7.3 After stabilizing the tube, an incision is made (in this case with a needle electrode) over the antimesosalpingeal border of the gestational site (courtesy of V. Gomel)

either omentum, peritoneum or other pelvic tissue. On completion of the procedure, the tube is usually left open to heal by secondary intention. It is important to note that it is unusual for the site of an ampullary ectopic pregnancy to develop either a fistula or obstruction at the site of treatment. This is thought perhaps to be due to the fact that many ampullary ectopic pregnancies do not develop within the lumen of the tube, but rather in the potential space between the serosa and muscularis layers of the tube (Figure 7.4).

For infundibular pregnancies in which the products of conception can be seen extruding from the tube at the time of diagnostic laparoscopy, the tissue products can be grasped and removed before completing the procedure. For infundibular eccyesis wherein no tissue is extruded, there is a tendency for practitioners to attempt to 'milk' the products of conception from the tube. This, however, is thought by many to cause damage to the tube and is therefore

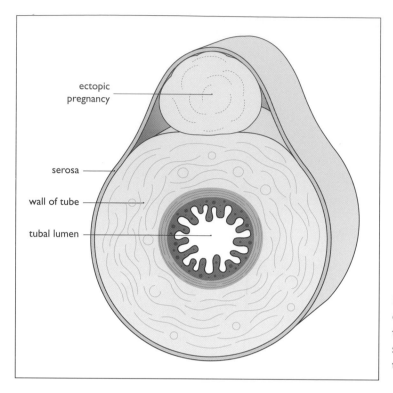

Figure 7.4 Many ampullary ectopic pregnancies develop in the potential space between the serosa and muscularis layers of the tube

to be discouraged. Alternatively, the infundibular ectopic pregnancy can be treated similarly to an ampullar ectopic pregnancy with an incision over the site of eccyesis. In such cases, the incision often extends to the fibriated end.

In contrast to ampullary ectopic pregnancies, isthmic ectopic pregnancies usually lie within the lumen of the Fallopian tube and thus, as with ampullary eccyeses, are treated by linear salpingostomy. It is therefore not surprising that these tubes have a relatively high rate of either occlusion or development of fistulas. Consequently, some surgeons recommend that isthmic ectopic pregnancies be treated by segmental resection. When the setting allows primary anastomosis of the tube (which requires microsurgical instrumentation, and staff familiar with its location and use), segmental resection presents a viable alternative. For the approximately 50% of patients who do not develop a fistula or obstruction, no further

surgical intervention is necessary whereas, for the other half of patients presenting with a fistula or obstruction, anastomosis can be performed later as if a segmental resection had initially been performed. This allows anastomosis to be carried out under controlled conditions when the tissue is not engorged due to pregnancy and when appropriate preparation for microsurgical procedures can be undertaken.

Patients with cornual or intramural ectopic pregnancies are a major source of concern because they often present late and with profound hemorrhage. Because of the propensity for bleeding and the large blood supply to this area, some surgeons do not recommend salpingostomy in these cases. Other surgeons may carry out salpingostomy, but with extensive coagulation of tissue, especially in patients who do not desire further conception.

For patients who do not desire future fertility or have a ruptured tube with a large

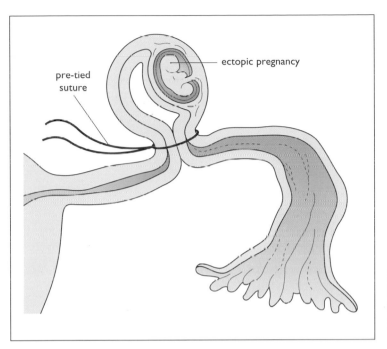

Figure 7.5 A pre-tied suture can be used to perform salpingectomy in cases where the ectopic pregnancy is discrete

ectopic pregnancy, salpingectomy may be the treatment of choice for the pregnancy. Two options are available – removal of the entire Fallopian tube or removal of a tubal segment. A variety of modalities are available for performing either partial or complete salpingectomy. If the ectopic pregnancy is discrete, a loose pre-tied suture is positioned to overlie the site of the tubal gestation (Figure 7.5). The tube is then elevated through the loop of the suture, which is then tightly cinched beneath the eccyesis to achieve hemostasis. This procedure can be repeated for a second or even third time, according to the surgeon's preferences. Care must be taken in placing the pre-tied suture to ensure that the tissue distal to the loop is excised and that there are no products of conception remaining in the tissue that is left behind. Furthermore, the pedicle needs to be of a sufficiently small size to allow the loop to be tightened to the point of hemostasis. This technique can also be used when the eccyesis is infundibular; in this case, the pre-tied suture is positioned over the fimbriated end

of the tube including the ectopic pregnancy.

An alternative to pre-tied sutures is the use of electrosurgery. The tube is grasped at one or more locations to allow coagulation of both the tube and the underlying blood vessels, which may also be incised (Figure 7.6). After coagulation is achieved, the tube can be incised at these sites. Subsequently, the mesosalpinx beneath the pregnancy can be coagulated to allow excision of the eccyesis (Figure 7.7).

A total salpingectomy can begin at either the fimbriated or the cornual portion of the Fallopian tube. If the procedure is to be initiated at the cornual end, the tube is coagulated at the site of its insertion into the uterus and incised. Alternatively, pre-tied suture loops (Endoloops™) can be placed over the cornual segment after division and the mesosalpinx subsequently incised, using a variety of techniques. One approach is to successively coagulate and incise the mesosalpinx, using a grasping instrument ipsilateral to the tube to retract the tube as each section is cut.

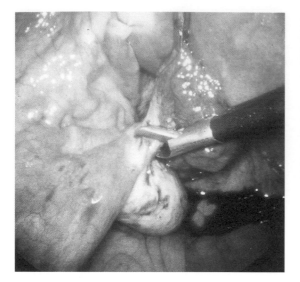

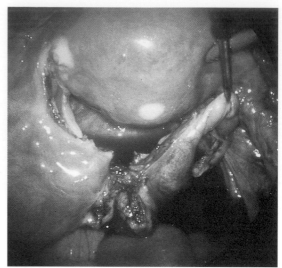

Figure 7.6 Electrodessication and transection of the tuboovarian ligament is performed prior to tubal excision (courtesy of V. Gomel)

Figure 7.7 Total excision of the tubal ectopic pregnancy is accomplished on complete division of the mesosalpinx (courtesy of V. Gomel)

An alternative is to use a linear cutting instrument which places multiple rows of staples while simultaneously incising between these rows of staples so that hemostasis is obtained both proximal and distal to the incision line. Linear cutters can be used to perform either partial or total salpingectomy. In the latter procedure, the tube is retracted medially to allow the linear cutter to 'hug' its mesenteric border. Before the cutter is 'fired', care must be taken to confirm that the infundibular pelvic vessels as well as the ureter will not be compromised.

When performing a partial salpingectomy, the surgeon must bear in mind the possibility of a repeat ectopic pregnancy in the remaining distal segment of the tube. This may occur if the contralateral tube is patent, thereby allowing the entrance of sperm into the peritoneal cavity. Patients should be made aware of this possibility and consider the use of some form of contraception until tubal anastomosis can be performed.

Following treatment of an ectopic pregnancy, whether by salpingostomy or salpingectomy, β-hCG titers should be followed at approximately weekly intervals until they fall to below the level of sensitivity for the assay. If the patient becomes symptomatic during the postoperative period or if titers rise, the physician should strongly suspect the possibility of a persistent ectopic pregnancy and make appropriate plans for either surgical or medical intervention. It has generally been accepted that, as long as the β-hCG titers continue to decrease, however slowly, and provided that the patients are considered to be responsible adults and remain asymptomatic, then only observation is necessary. However, this decision should take into consideration whether the patient lives alone, the time it would take for the patient to get to hospital in case of an emergency, and the availability of other healthcare providers.

8 Myomectomy

Uterine leiomyomas

Uterine leiomyomas are found in a relatively large proportion of women, approaching 30 35% in many series. The symptomatology, however, varies greatly and many leiomyomas remain asymptomatic. In some patients, leiomyomas may contribute to a variety of clinical syndromes that involve irregular bleeding, pelvic pain, infertility and distortion of the surrounding organs, including the bladder and bowel. This wide variation in symptoms is a reflection of the many factors, such as size, vascular supply, and location on (anterior wall, cervical, fundal or posterior wall) and within (serosal, intramural or submucosal) the uterus, associated with uterine leiomyomas (Figure 8.1).

Uterine leiomyomas are often identified at the time of pelvic examination. On palpation, the uterus often feels enlarged and may have, in addition, an irregular contour. However, intracavitary myomas and some that are intramural are frequently missed during pelvic examination. Further characterization of the size and location of fibroids can be achieved by a variety of imaging modalities. Probably the most commonly used modality at present is ultrasonography, in particular, transvaginal ultrasonography. Ultrasound allows identification of the number, size and location of the fibroids. However, on occasions, it may be difficult to distinguish fibroids from other pelvic structures or masses. Intracavitary uterine leiomyomas can be diagnosed by either hysterosalpingography, sonohysterography

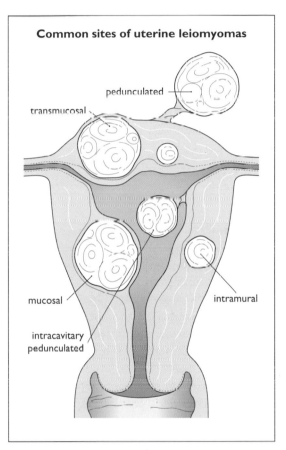

Figure 8.1 Uterine leiomyomas may be located at a variety of sites on or within the uterus

and / or hysteroscopy. This is particularly important in women presenting with infertility. Although many theories have been postulated to explain how myomas may contribute to infertility, only a few have become accepted, including the presence of myomas in the uterine cavity and those which cause tubal obstruction. The mechanism(s) by which myomas within the uterine cavity contribute to infertility has not yet been established, but theories include:

(1) The endometrial surface overlying the myoma possesses a poor blood supply and, thus, an impaired potential for nidation;

(2) A grossly enlarged cavity necessitates a longer distance for the sperm to travel before reaching the upper reproductive tract;

(3) A pseudoinflammatory response becomes established within the cavity; and

(4) There is contrecoup damage of the endometrial surface on the uterine wall opposite the myoma.

Recently, transvaginal ultrasound (particularly if performed concomitantly with instillation of fluid into the uterus), computed tomography (CT) and magnetic resonance imaging (MRI) have been used for the further assessment of uterine myomas. The major disadvantage of these techniques is the cost associated with their performance. In addition, with CT scans, there is a small amount of radiation exposure to the female gonads and reproductive tract. However, these modalities all have the potential to provide highly reliable clinical information. In particular, the use of MRI with image-intensifying body coils has at times allowed the differentiation of structures and diagnostic information that was otherwise not available with the other modalities. This has included the identification of blood vessels in the stalk of a pedunculated myoma, the capacity to distinguish a broad ligament myoma from other adnexal structures, and the differentiation of benign from malignant uterine myomas.

Uterine myomas may contribute to the symptoms they cause in a variety of ways, including pelvic pain and irregular bleeding. Pelvic pain may be due to the effects of the enlarged uterus compressing surrounding organs such as the bowel and bladder or it may be the result of a myoma outgrowing its blood supply, resulting in ischemia and sometimes infarction as a result of torsion which, in turn, can result in acute ischemia associated with excruciating pelvic pain. Irregular bleeding in patients with myomas is thought to most likely represent irregular shedding of the endometrial surface overlying the myoma that is specific to that portion of the uterine cavity. The shedding may be due to mechanical factors or to variations in the blood supply (and therefore hormonal exposure) to these areas.

Options for treatment

The mere presence of uterine myomas is not in itself an indication for surgical treatment. In the absence of symptoms, observation may be all that is required. However, when symptoms are present, the patient should be evaluated for possible treatment by either medical or surgical means. Medical therapy of uterine myomas is primarily based on the fact that, as fibroids are estrogen-dependent tumors, the reduction of estrogenic effects (either by decreasing estrogen levels or increasing opposition to estrogen effects) should reduce tumor size.

Short-term medical therapy is often effective in reducing the size of uterine leiomyomas although, following cessation of therapy, myomas often regain their pretreatment size. Thus, medical therapy is frequently used as a delaying technique, the goal of which may be to allow an anemic patient time to bolster her blood count (and potentially to bank blood prior to surgery) or, in perimenopausal women, to shrink myomas sufficiently so as to allow the patient to remain relatively asymptomatic until the onset of menopause, thereby obviating the need for surgical therapy.

At present, the most commonly used medical therapy is probably with gonadotropin-releasing hormone (GnRH) analogues. With such treatment, myomas often reach their least size within 3–4 months of starting therapy. Because of concerns regarding osteoporosis and other estrogen-deficiency syndromes, GnRH therapy is usually limited to 6 months. In future, the introduction of add-back regimens in which low doses of estrogen or progestin are given concomitantly with GnRH analogues may allow the possibility of achieving the beneficial effects of GnRH analogues for longer periods of time without the potential risk of osteoporosis and other conditions. This may allow the prolonged use of medical therapy for the treatment of uterine fibroids.

An additional potential benefit of preoperative GnRH therapy is the reduction of preoperative blood loss, which may make the dissection easier to perform. Although several studies have suggested that blood loss may be reduced, the reproducibility and clinical significance of the benefits achieved are as yet uncertain. There is even greater controversy regarding the effect of GnRH analogue therapy on ease of dissection as many surgeons believe that the appropriate plane for dissection is more difficult to identify following analogue treatment, thereby rendering the procedure more difficult to perform.

Uterine leiomyosarcomas

Although uterine leiomyosarcomas are rare, they remain a possibility so that the question then remains of how to distinguish a benign from a malignant myoma. Specific guidelines that are totally accurate are not available, although malignancy should be strongly suspected in myomas that undergo rapid growth and enlargement. MRI helps in making these distinctions on the basis of the consistency and appearance of the myoma itself. Suspicion should also be raised when a myoma fails to diminish with GnRH therapy and particularly when a myoma increases in size with GnRH. In patients with multiple myomas, it is often especially difficult to follow each separate myoma to assess whether any are increasing in size. In a recent review of a 10-year history of leiomyosarcomas at the Yale – New Haven Hospital, it was found that 95% of subjects with uterine leiomyosarcoma had malignancy in the largest myoma. This suggests that it is particularly important to follow the largest myoma to determine any changes in size with GnRH analogue therapy when monitoring of all myomas is not possible. Although this cannot uniformly identify all leiomyosarcomas, this experience suggests that such a compromise will be helpful.

A further concern raised regarding the medical therapy of leiomyomas prior to surgical therapy is whether modulation of the hormonal milieu has any effect on the histological characteristics of myomas so as to increase the difficulty in distinguishing a benign from a malignant uterine leiomyosarcoma. This issue was recently evaluated in women receiving GnRH therapy. The study assessed 10 different histological criteria, including the degree of vascularity, classification and cellular reactivity, in myomas removed from patients who had either received or not received treatment with GnRH analogues. On comparison of these two patient groups, there were apparently no significant differences among the histological criteria. Furthermore, when assessing myomas which had decreased in size with those which had not decreased with GnRH therapy, no histological differences were identified. Thus, presurgical therapy with a GnRH analogue is apparently not likely to make the job of the pathologist significantly more difficult.

Surgical therapy

Uterine leiomyomas can be surgically treated by either hysterectomy or myomectomy. Although there is anecdotal evidence that difficulties encountered during myomectomy frequently lead to modification of the surgical plan (including conversion to hysterectomy or non-autologous blood transfusion), the frequency of such occurrences is apparently low. When patients desire fertility, hysterectomy is clearly not a desirable option. Also, there are women who no longer desire childbearing, but who want to preserve their uterus. In these cases, although hysterectomy can be discussed as an option, they often choose myomectomy even when they are aware of the high frequency with which myomas may recur. This is particularly so in women with multiple myomas rather than a single isolated myoma. Previous studies have shown that patients with multiple myomas have a higher rate of recurrence which may, however, not represent true recurrence, but rather the growth of small myomas not identified and / or treated during the initial operation. For this reason, at the time of myomectomy, it is recommended that all 'seedling' myomas be removed.

For women who wish to preserve their uterus, myomectomy can be performed at the time of laparotomy, laparoscopy or hysteroscopy. Hysteroscopy is carried out in cases where the myoma extends into the uterine cavity and can be accomplished by a variety of modalities, including the resectoscope and fiber lasers (see *A Manual of Clinical Hysteroscopy* by R.F. Valle). The goal of hysteroscopic therapy is to excise the myoma down to the level of the surrounding myometrium. This is often performed under laparoscopic guidance particularly when the practitioner has had little experience with this operation or the myoma is large. However, with this treatment, the portion of the myoma that was intramural is often left behind to possibly regrow and redevelop, although such an occurrence is uncommon. On occasions, patients have reported tissue loss, which is thought to represent spontaneous expulsion of the residual intramural portion of the myoma.

Subserosal, pedunculated and intramural myomas are more commonly treated by either abdominal laparotomy or laparoscopy. Surgical goals of an abdominal approach include total excision of the myoma(s) followed by restoration of the integrity of the myometrium to allow subsequent pregnancy. Considerable attention is paid to closure of the serosal surface of the uterus to minimize postoperative adhesion development. In general, it is preferable to keep both the number and size of serosal incisions to a minimum; thus, lateral dissection from one myoma cavity to the site of an adjacent myoma is preferable to making a second serosal incision, although this may not always be possible. If the uterine cavity is to be entered while removing a myoma, some surgeons suggest removing the myoma from the opposite wall after traversing the uterine cavity. However, when the cavity is not to be entered as part of the procedure, entry for the sole purpose of transcavity treatment of another myoma is generally to be avoided. In such cases, a second serosal incision is more usual. If possible, incisions in the posterior uterine surface should be avoided as these are the areas most likely to be involved in tubal and ovarian adhesions, thereby limiting fertility. In addition, it is preferable that incisions avoid the uterine cornua, as this will minimize the likelihood of an inci-

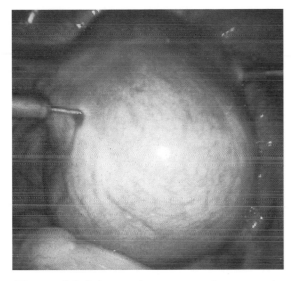

Figure 8.2 Subserosal injection of vasopressin reduces the vascular supply in preparation for removal of the myoma (courtesy of G.F. Scarselli)

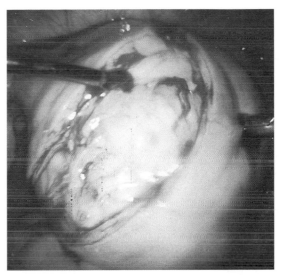

Figure 8.3 A harmonic scalpel dissecting hook is used to resect the myometrium for complete exposure of the myoma (courtesy of G.F. Scarselli)

sion extending towards the tube and avoid placement of a stitch (to establish hemostasis and / or restore the myometrium wall) which may result in distortion and damage to the intramural segment of the Fallopian tube.

At the time of laparotomy, a variety of techniques can be used to reduce blood loss, including: injection of synthetic vasopressin (20 units in 100 mL of saline; Figure 8.2); placing a tourniquet around the lower uterine segment; or positioning bulldog clamps over the infundibular pelvic ligaments. Indeed, other techniques can also be used as greater efficacy with any of these techniques has not been demonstrated. In general, the incision is made over the myoma, whether subserosal or intramural. Dissection is carried down to the level of the capsule, using either sharp dissection, electrosurgical or laser techniques (Figure 8.3). Enucleation of the myoma usually consists of a combination of blunt and sharp dissection, and is facilitated by putting

tension on the myoma either by placing a large suture through the myoma, or grasping the myoma with towel clips or with a corkscrew-type instrument. Dissection is carried out around the myoma. Occasionally, large vascular pedicles can be identified and tied although, in other cases, it may be difficult to identify the specific vessels leading to the myoma. After removing the myoma and confirming that there is no myoma lying adjacent, the leiomyoma cavity is closed with sutures, beginning at the deepest point of the cavity (Figure 8.4).

Depending on the size of the myoma, a single or multiple layers may be involved and, depending on the redundancy of the serosal surfaces, small amounts of myometrium may be trimmed away. The serosal surface is then closed, using a relatively fine suture with low tissue reactivity and techniques such as imbrication of the sutures to minimize the amount of suture exposure to the serosa in an attempt to minimize the development of adhesions.

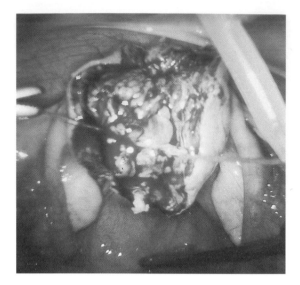

Figure 8.4 After removal of the myoma, the deep portions of the defect are closed with sutures (courtesy of G.F. Scarselli)

Small seedling myomas may be vaporized by electrosurgery or laser, or excised during multiple myomectomy. However, in patients not otherwise undergoing uterine surgery and if the seedling myomas are asymptomatic, these may be left untreated because the risk of these seedlings causing infertility may be lower than the likelihood of postoperative adhesion development following their surgical treatment. When these small myomas are treated, the resultant defects can usually be easily closed or left open. In either situation, obtaining hemostasis is of paramount importance.

Recently, the laparoscopic treatment of uterine leiomyomas has received increased attention, although the role of laparoscopy in the treatment of myomas remains unclear. With pedunculated myomas, laparoscopy may be effective in their excision, although difficulty often arises in the subsequent removal of large myomas from the abdominal cavity. Removal may entail a posterior colpotomy incision or morcellation of the myoma into pieces that fit through either a

laparoscopic trocar sleeve or an enlarged abdominal wall incision. The surgical technique employed to dissect free subserosal and intramural myomas is similar to that used at the time of laparotomy. The myoma is grasped and placed on tension to facilitate its dissection.

A major question, however, is the reason for removal of uterine myomas. Because myomectomy can be performed laparoscopically is not a good reason to perform the procedure. At present, the number of cases selected for laparoscopic therapy is similar to the number selected for laparotomy.

Whereas experience with laparoscopic myomectomy suggests that intraoperative and postoperative bleeding is apparently not a major problem, one issue which remains unclarified is the capacity to restore the integrity of the myometrium with laparoscopy. This issue is particularly important in women desiring fertility. In a series of 24 patients who had undergone laparoscopic intramural myomectomy, 6 (25%) subsequently developed a fistula between the uterine and abdominal cavities. This suggests that the greater the difficulty of the operation at laparoscopy, the fewer the attempts to close the defect in a manner analogous to that achieved at laparotomy. Even in those patients without a fistula, the defect left behind in the myometrium with laparoscopy may predispose to uterine rupture during subsequent pregnancy. Thus, in patients desiring future fertility, removal of large subserosal intramural myomas may be placing the patient at an increased risk during a subsequent gestation. However, in future, with the development of other approaches and better suture techniques, reestablishing myometrial integrity may cease to be a problem.

Recently, several surgeons have suggested an alternative to the excision of myomas. Using either an electrosurgical needle or cryosurgical device, the surgeon attempts to destroy the vasculature of the myoma, thereby causing it to regress in size. The efficacy of this new approach compared with other techniques, as well as the long-term outcome, remain to be established.

A further issue is the treatment of the uterine serosal surface at the time of laparotomy and laparoscopy particularly in women desiring fertility. When the incision lies on the posterior uterine surface in the proximity of the tubes and ovaries, the question yet to be answered is whether closure of the serosal incision results in a higher incidence of postoperative adhesion development.

9 Adhesiolysis

Adhesions are a major contributing factor to infertility when they involve the Fallopian tubes and ovaries, and contribute significantly to pelvic pain. They are the leading non-cancerous cause of bowel obstruction. Consequently, the lysis of adhesions frequently represents a major procedure for the pelvic surgeon although, on occasions, adhesiolysis is the initial stage of a procedure to allow treatment of other pathology that may involve other organs in the pelvis.

It is important to realize that adhesion development after pelvic surgery is a common occurrence. In a recent collaborative study involving 68 women undergoing operative laparoscopy, it was noted that 66 (97%) had pelvic adhesions at the time of a second-look procedure; adhesion development occurred despite the use of a variety of different operative approaches. Thus, laparoscopic surgery is not a panacea for postoperative adhesion development.

Of perhaps even greater interest was the observation that, on recurrence, the adhesions were not always thick and vascular but were, in some cases, fine, thin and filmy (like Saran Wrap®) prior to adhesiolysis. Furthermore, adhesions appear to recur in patients irrespective of the amount of adhesions initially present. As a result, those patients who had minimal adhesion development at the time of initial operation were subsequently identified to be among those who had the greatest worsening of adhesions. Thus, there continues to be a great need for modification of surgical techniques, instruments and equipment, and the use of adjuvants to further reduce the development of postoperative adhesions.

Probably the most important means by which a surgeon may reduce postoperative adhesion development is to pay careful attention to the surgical techniques employed. Whenever possible, surgeons should strive to follow the basic guidelines of gynecological microsurgery (Table 9.1), although there are several caveats. First, the processes of both visualization and surgery as well as the placing of traction and countertraction invariably involve the manipulation of tissues. However, such involvement should be as atraumatic as possible to minimize damage to the peritoneal serosa. One method of achieving this is by grasping and manipulating only the tissue to be excised rather than the tissue to be left behind. Another approach is to use atraumatic graspers whenever possible. During laparotomy, the packs intended for use should be dampened and positioned such that trauma to serosal surfaces is minimized.

Although attaining hemostasis is of paramount importance, the means by which

Table 9.1 Classical tenets of gynecological microsurgery

Minimize tissue-handling
Achieve meticulous hemostasis
Avoid the introduction of foreign bodies
Use an appropriate magnification
Use fine non-reactive sutures
Avoid tissue dessication

hemostasis is achieved may have significant effects on subsequent adhesion development. If hemostasis is obtained by tying off large tissue pedicles, the tissue distal to the suture must eventually be resorbed and may become adhesiogenic. Similarly, if large areas are devitalized by extensive electrocoagulation, the healing process may be adhesiogenic. Thus, sites of bleeding should be identified as precisely as possible and hemostasis obtained with as little resultant devitalization of tissue as possible.

An additional tenet which is not included in Table 9.1, but which is often raised, concerns the precision with which approximation of the tissue planes is carried out. Although this issue has long been included among the basic tenets of gynecological microsurgery, there is growing uncertainty as to its accuracy, particularly when vital structures are not involved. In a variety of animal studies, the results suggest that adhesion formation is similar or even greater at sites which are reperitonealized rather than left open. Although the data in clinical studies have not been collected from well-designed studies, the results tend to confirm the animal data. Thus, this may well represent an area of change in clinical practice.

In many ways, the procedure in laparoscopic adhesiolysis is similar to adhesiolysis at laparotomy. The same general principles apply: there must be adequate visualization of the adhesions to be lysed (Figure 9.1); and traction and countertraction need to be developed to facilitate dissection. With laparoscopy, traction and countertraction are achieved by the use of instruments in other ports and by manipulation of the uterine probe (Figure 9.2). Thus, for procedures involving the right adnexa, the uterus is deviated to the left. Similarly, for procedures involving the posterior cul-de-sac, the uterus is anteverted toward the bladder.

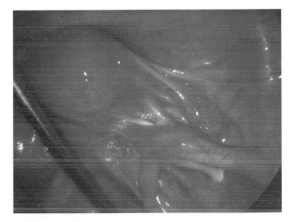

Figure 9.1 Tuboovarian and tubouterine adhesions, and adhesions on the ovary extending to the pelvic wall (courtesy of R.A. Steiner, from Cosmi EV, ed. *FIGO Gynecological Endoscopy Slide Series*, 1996)

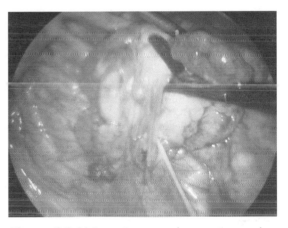

Figure 9.2 Using scissors and a uterine probe, adhesions are stretched and divided one layer at a time parallel to the organ involved (in this case, the Fallopian tube) (courtesy of V. Gomel)

As with procedures performed at laparotomy, tissue planes are often identifiable with laparoscopy. In general, it is preferable to excise, rather than incise, adhesions and to expose as little of the surface area of the pelvic organs and peritoneum as possible. Thus, as a general rule, it may be safer to leave a portion of an adhesion in place rather than risk damage to the visceral or parietal peritoneum.

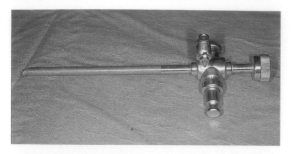

Figure 9.3 This specially designed trocar sleeve for use as a backstop for a CO_2 laser, has a sandblasted surface and may also be used for irrigation

When a CO_2 laser is to be used, consideration must be given to the backstop to be placed behind the adhesions. This may be a specially designed trocar sleeve (with a sandblasted surface; Figure 9.3) which can be used for irrigation as well. In the process of lysing adhesions to the anterior abdominal wall or posterior surface of the uterus, the pelvis may be filled with irrigating solutions to minimize the likelihood of damage to the sigmoid colon. Although the CO_2 laser is an instrument frequently used by many surgeons, there is no evidence that its use (or the use, for that matter, of any other type of laser) either reduces the development of postoperative adhesions or improves pregnancy outcome compared with other techniques and modalities. Thus, the use of a laser is solely according to the preferences of the surgeon. The patient should not be counseled that the use of the laser *per se* will improve the efficacy of the procedure.

10 Endometriosis

Endometriosis is defined as the presence of endometrial glands and stroma at sites outside of the uterus. The most common locations are the dependent portions of the pelvis, including the posterior cul-de-sac, pelvic side walls, sigmoid colon and ovaries. However, endometriosis can also be identified at other sites throughout the pelvis and abdominal cavity and, less frequently, at distant sites throughout the body such as the lungs or brain.

The etiology of endometriosis is, as yet, unknown. Suggested theories include Sampson's theory of retrograde menstruation, which is the most generally accepted possibility. However, other theories include celomic metaplasia, hematogenous or lymphatic dissemination and direct spread (for example, via episiotomy or Cesarean section incisions), and all attempt to explain the locations at which endometriosis has been identified.

Classical endometriosis has been described as purplish-black lesions involving the peritoneum and ovary. Recently, however, it has been shown that endometriosis has a number of other appearances as well (Figures 10.1–10.3). Indeed, it has been suggested that the classical purplish-black lesions are those which have already run their course whereas other endometriotic implants, appearing as clear blebs, or reddish or yellowish lesions, may be those that are still active. These active lesions may produce prostaglandins and other molecules with biological activity that may be responsible, in part, for some of the deleterious

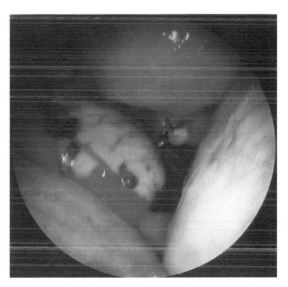

Figure 10.1 Purplish-black puckered superficial lesions of endometriosis on the right ovary (courtesy of T. Gürgan)

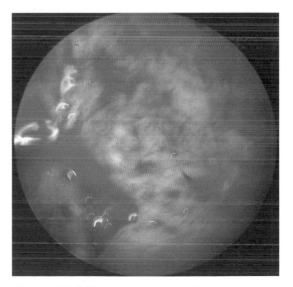

Figure 10.2 Flame-like lesions of endometriosis on the pelvic wall (courtesy of T. Gürgan)

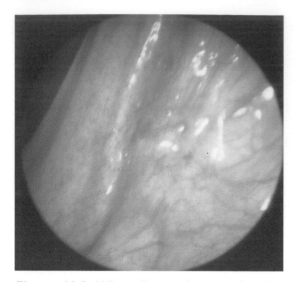

Figure 10.3 White fibrotic lesions of endometriosis on the pelvic wall (courtesy of T. Gürgan)

consequences of endometriosis, such as pelvic pain, infertility and the development of adhesions.

Endometriosis can also present as masses within the ovary (so-called ovarian endometrioma) or in the soft tissue of the pelvis as, for example, rectovaginal nodules that are often palpated during examination of the rectovaginal septum. A full description of the etiology of endometriosis, and its diagnosis, identification and consequences, are beyond the scope of this book. For further information, the reader is referred to the selected bibliography.

Small implants of endometriosis can be treated in a variety of ways and, at present, there are no definitive findings to suggest that one treatment method is better than the others. However, regardless of the method selected, results are likely to be superior if the lesions are totally eradicated. One commonly used treatment approach is fulguration of the lesions by electrosurgery, using either unipolar or bipolar electrosurgical instrumentation. Unipolar electrosurgery (see Chapter 3) is associated with a greater depth of penetration and greater degrees of tissue destruction than is bipolar electrosurgery. The end-point with this modality is usually blanching of the peritoneum involved with the lesion. It is essential, however, that the surgeon be aware of other anatomical structures in the vicinity of the endometriotic implant and, thus, modulate the use of energy to minimize the potential for damage to adjacent structures.

When CO_2 laser energy is used on the pelvic side walls, the end-point is usually when normal-looking tissue beneath the site of the endometriotic implant is reached. Because of the suggestion that endometriotic implants may tunnel beneath the peritoneum from the point of the lesion seen on the surface, it may be considered good practice to treat the peritoneum immediately surrounding the area of the lesion as well as the lesion itself. This should minimize the possibility of leaving a portion of the endometriotic implant behind. However, this practice should be based on the experience of the surgeon and the proximity of the surrounding vital structures. The treatment of endometriotic lesions with argon and KTP–532 lasers is similar to that with the CO_2 laser, although there is a tendency towards greater tissue penetration. Some surgeons also use the Nd:YAG laser (particularly with sapphire and sculptured tips) to treat endometriotic implants.

An alternative to fulguration or vaporization of the lesions is excision. Some surgeons suggest excision of the peritoneum surrounding individual lesions because of peritoneal extension as described above with wide vaporization. The peritoneum is incised with either scissors or other modality, and then grasped and elevated to allow excision of the lesion from the underlying connective tissue by sharp dissection, electrosurgery

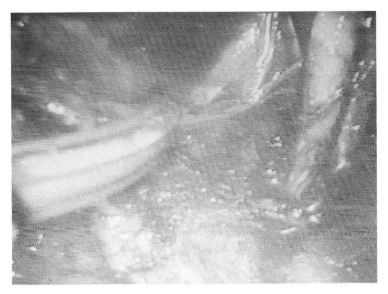

Figure 10.4 Endometriotic plaque is stripped away from the ureter and uterosacral ligament by sharp dissection and electrosurgery (courtesy of O.M. Petrucco)

(Figure 10.4) or laser. Such a technique has been used to document the various appearances of endometriosis other than the typical bluish-black lesion. As an aid to the pathological diagnosis of endometriosis, presenting the pathologist with a small specimen is advantageous as the tissue that is apparently endometriotic can then be sectioned for histological examination. When the pathologist receives a large block of tissue, there is a risk that those parts not suspected of endometriosis may, in fact, be sent for sectioning and histological assessment, thereby resulting in undiagnosed endometriosis.

It is becoming increasingly recognized that endometriosis may infiltrate the tissues beneath the peritoneum. In such cases, it is important to treat the subperitoneal disease as well, although this may involve more extensive dissection that may exceed the capabilities of many endoscopic surgeons. Nevertheless, it is important to document these infiltrating lesions even if the surgeon is not able to treat them surgically so that the patient can be appropriately informed and postoperative medical therapy considered.

Although endometriotic lesions involving the peritoneum of the bladder or

bowel can be treated endoscopically, such lesions have an immediate potential to cause damage to these organs. Injuries may be identified at the time of the surgical procedure or they may develop postoperatively after many days. Thus, the treatment of lesions involving these and other vital tissues requires a greater degree of experience and skill particularly in cases where the lesions are larger or more infiltrative.

Occasionally, advanced endoscopic surgery is performed which involves entry into the bladder or bowel for removal of full-thickness endometriotic lesions with subsequent endoscopic repair. Clearly, this is beyond the capabilities of practitioners who are beginners at endoscopic surgery. Nevertheless, it is important to note that, in patients thought to have pathology involving the bowel, preoperative exploratory bowel surgery is appropriate because of the possibility of unintended entry into the bowel. If more extensive disease is encountered, the surgeon should be comfortable with the decision to proceed to laparotomy as part of a planned (or unplanned) conversion because of the pathology or complications encountered. Patients should be counseled

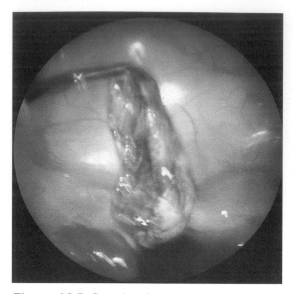

Figure 10.5 Capsule of an endometrioma cyst following total cystectomy (courtesy of T. Gürgan)

when such a conversion is considered to be likely.

Some surgeons treat extensive endometriosis involving the posterior cul-de-sac by extensive dissection of the peritoneum throughout the cul-de-sac. Because of the large number of vital structures encountered by such dissection, this procedure should not be performed by the relatively inexperienced endoscopic surgeon. The value of such extensive dissection remains controversial.

Small spots of endometriosis involving the ovarian surface can be vaporized or fulgurated as has been described for endometriotic spots on the peritoneum, and ovarian endometriomas can be similarly treated. Although, by tradition, endometriomas are considered to be cysts which develop within ovarian tissue, an alternative hypothesis has recently been suggested. An endometrioma may develop from surface implants with overlying adhesions which stretch from the margins of the implant and come into contact with normal ovarian cortex. If bleeding occurs at these implants, the adhesion traps the blood and prevents it from spreading diffusely throughout the abdominal cavity. If the volume of blood is sufficiently large so as not to be dissipated, it will collect at that site, thus forming an endometrioma. Pressure causes the endometrioma to appear to invaginate into the ovary.

Small endometriomas can be opened by an incision in the ovarian cortex and the cavity fulgurated or vaporized. With larger endometriomas, this technique becomes less effective as vaporization of large endometriomas produces large plumes of smoke, which may impede performance of the procedure. Perhaps even more important is the damage to the surrounding tissues caused by the heat.

The first step in the treatment of ovarian endometriomas is incision and evacuation of the old hemorrhagic material. The ovarian cavity can then be examined to confirm the presence of endometrioma before commencing with treatment. (A discussion of the determination of benign from malignant ovarian masses is beyond the scope of this chapter. The reader is referred to recent publications concerning this important issue.) Larger endometriomas may be treated by stripping out the cavity lining, a procedure that may be facilitated by the placement of relaxing incisions to help initiate a plane of dissection. Using multiple graspers, the normal ovarian tissue and the endometrioma capsule can be dissected apart. Residual pieces of endometrioma capsule can then be vaporized or fulgurated. Alternatively, some surgeons excise the entire endometrioma (Figure 10.5) although, unless great care is taken, this may often result in loss of normal ovarian tissue as well.

The treatment of endometriosis is complicated due to a number of reasons.

First, histological evaluation of resected endometriomas has sometimes revealed that the tissue was, in fact, a corpus luteum cyst. Distinguishing between these two entities can be difficult even for the very experienced surgeon. Second, endometriosis involving the reproductive organs can also involve organs of the genitourinary and gastrointestinal tracts, necessitating treatment of these sites. However, laparoscopic resection of infiltrating endometriosis involving the bladder, ureters and bowel may be beyond the expertise of most gynecologists. Some may be willing to go only as far as to remove an appendix which contains endometriosis (as many gynecologists are trained to perform appendectomies at laparotomy).

There are a number of approaches for performing laparoscopic appendectomy; only one option is described here. The mesoappendix and its blood vessels can be 'skeletonized' off the appendix, with hemostasis achieved by electrocautery or another modality. A series of three suture loops can then be placed at the base of the appendix, leaving a space to transect the appendix between the second and third ties from the cecum. The suture from the first and second loops is cut whereas a long end is left on the third tie. The appendix is then cut and the free end manipulated by the long suture to allow removal of the appendix through a trocar sleeve. After confirming hemostasis, some surgeons may choose to cauterize the cut edge of the appendix; others may simply bury it by oversewing the adjacent cecum.

Third, endometriosis with or without adhesions frequently results in pelvic pain. Thus, in addition to treating the endometriotic lesions and adhesions, some surgeons believe there may be some benefit from procedures which remove afferent neurons. Two procedures performed for this purpose are transection of the uterosacral ligaments

and presacral neurectomy. The value of each is controversial, although it is generally agreed that the patients who are likely to benefit from these procedures are women with central (not adnexal) pain. Several procedures for uterosacral transection for pelvic pain have been described and claim to result in benefit for approximately 70% of patients. Most of these studies, however, lacked a control group and, thus, any benefit may in part represent a placebo effect. There has been one randomized study (involving only around 20 patients) where no pathology was noted in patients at laparoscopy. These patients were then blindly randomized to receive either transection or placebo. Postoperatively, although all patients initially reported a benefit, at the time of follow-up 1 year later, only the treated group reported a reduction in pain.

An important consideration when performing this procedure is the anatomical relationship of the uterosacral ligament to the uterine and ovarian vessels, and to the ureter. These structures normally lie close to the insertion of the uterosacral ligament into the cervix; thus, energy dispersion to these structures must be considered and the procedure appropriately performed so as to transect the ligament with minimal lateral tissue injury. Such considerations would tend to lead the surgeon to transect the uterosacral ligaments at a distance somewhat removed from the cervix. However, some of the nerve fibers are likely to diverge as they become more distal, and thus the procedure may be less complete. In addition to transection of the uterosacral ligaments, some surgeons also advocate treating the area between the uterosacral ligaments along the posterior of the cervix.

An alternative therapy for central pain is presacral neurectomy which can be performed either at laparotomy or laparoscopy. As with transection of the uterosacral ligaments, the efficacy of this procedure is controversial. The peritoneum is incised caudal to the sacral promontory to isolate the tissue which contains nerve fibers which run from the right common iliac vein to the mesentary of the sigmoid colon on the left. A section of this tissue is excised to separate the nerve fibers. Most operations using this procedure were conducted at laparotomy, although many advanced endoscopic surgeons perform it laparoscopically. It appears that presacral neurectomy may be helpful in reducing pelvic pain in carefully selected patients.

It might be expected, from the regions of the nerves being cut, that transection of the uterosacral ligaments or presacral neurectomy could contribute to bladder dysfunction, constipation, altered orgasmic response and / or uterine prolapse. Where these responses have been described, the extent to which they complicate these procedures has remained unproven.

11 Distal tubal surgery

Distal tubal surgery generally involves those patients with distal tubal disease who have either total or partial tubal obstruction, each of which is often accompanied by adhesions with or without endometriosis. If these are present, it can be assumed that, at the time of distal tubal surgery, the tubes are completely freed from any surrounding adhesions and the implants of endometriosis treated.

Before undergoing distal tubal surgery, all patients should be assessed, usually by either hysterosalpingogram or prior laparoscopy with chromotubation and / or at the time of surgery by chromotubation to confirm tubal status. In tubes that are partially obstructed, the site(s) of blockage can also be determined to allow all to be appropriately treated. Similarly, if the distal tube obstruction is complete, important information can be gathered, including the degree of tubal distention and the site at which to open the tube.

On the basis of the preoperative information, the surgeon should discuss the options for therapy with the patient, including treatment at laparoscopy and at laparotomy, and the alternatives, mainly the different forms of assisted-reproduction technology. Decisions should be based on the individual characteristics of the given patient and her desires. Although it is clearly possible to treat partial or complete distal tubal obstruction laparoscopically, in my opinion, laparotomy remains the gold standard, particularly for cases with more extensive partial obstruction or complete distal tubal obstruction. However, not all surgeons agree on this point; some believe that, if a patient cannot be treated laparoscopically, then that patient should be entered into an assisted-reproduction technology program (for example, *in vitro* fertilization).

Neosalpingostomy and fimbrioplasty

In terms of terminology, a neosalpingostomy here refers to the creation of a new opening in a previously totally obstructed tube and a fimbrioplasty refers to the reconstruction of the distal end of a Fallopian tube that was previously partially obstructed. However, patient prognoses vary widely even within these categories. Prognostic factors for distal tubal obstruction include the concomitant pathology, size of the hydrosalpinx, wall thickness and the presence or absence of internal rugae: large, thin-walled, smooth tubes carry a poor prognosis (Figure 11.1).

The difficulty in counseling a patient who is soon to undergo fimbrioplasty is related to the wide variation in tubal disease seen in earlier reports describing the outcomes of fimbrioplasty in various series. The range of variation extends from tubes with a pinpoint opening and extensive damage to the tubal mucosa to those with only slight fibrial adhesions and totally normal tubal mucosa. Thus, the expected outcomes in series of fimbrioplasty may, in fact, cover a wide variety of patients, including those with only a pinpoint tubal opening to those undergoing adhesiolysis alone.

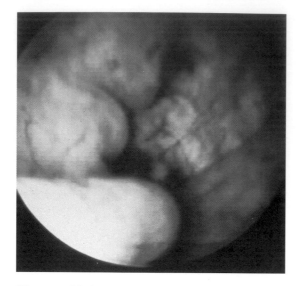

Figure 11.1 Endosalpinx showing loss of ampullar mucosal folds (methylene blue) (courtesy of G.F. Scarselli)

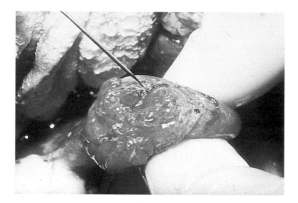

Figure 11.2 A unipolar cautery needle is used to enlarge the tubal ostium at laparotomy (courtesy of A.H. DeCherney)

To perform neosalpingostomy, a three- or four-puncture technique is used and instruments are placed in the vagina or cervix for instillation of dye or for tubal distention. Following tubal distention, the 'dimple' is visualized at the distal end of the tube which represents the site for the initial incision into the Fallopian tube (Figure 11.2). The modality selected (scissors, electro-surgical instrument or laser) is a matter of personal preference. Using grasping instru-

ments, the tissue on either side of the ostium is grasped and the opening further increased by a linear incision. When the opening is sufficiently large, the tubal serosa can be partially everted and / or an endoscope placed within the tube to examine the mucosa. Subsequent incisions in the tubal serosa are then attempted along areas of scarring which appear to have little or no normal fimbria so that extension of the incisions spare the normal fimbria as much as possible. Usually, around three to five cruciate incisions are made, emanating from the dimple, the number depending on the size of the tube, amount of scarring and tubal anatomy. In patients with a narrow hydro-salpinx, a single incision may be made along the entire antimesenteric border of the tube. The length of the cruciate incisions varies according to the anatomy, but is usually 1–3 cm in length. After creating the opening, the newly freed ends of the tube may be fastened in such a position as to maintain the opening. This can be achieved by either suturing or use of what has become known as the Bruhat technique, in which low levels of energy (either laser or electrosurgical) are applied along the serosal edges of the tube, thereby coagulating the serosal surfaces to result in eversion of the newly created tubal flaps. Some surgeons do not attempt to further maintain patency beyond making the cruciate incisions.

Pinpoint openings of the Fallopian tube are treated laparoscopically similarly to tubes that have total distal occlusion. However, tubes which undergo fimbrio-plasty often have other anatomical abnormal-ities, such as intrafimbrial adhesions which may be more vascular than usually seen with adhesions. These are best treated by incision, using a technique which produces minimal bleeding and, thus, minimal coagulation. If a laser or electrosurgical instrument is used, care should be taken to ensure that lateral

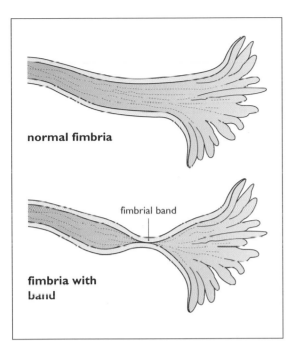

normal fimbria

fimbrial band

fimbria with band

Figure 11.3 A fimbrial band in the tube

and deep thermal energy spread is kept to a minimum.

Fimbrial bands

Another often encountered pathology involving the distal Fallopian tube is the apparent circumferential thickening, normally within approximately 1 cm of the distal end of the tube, called a fimbrial band (Figure 11.3). Identification of fimbrial bands is made by the presence of tubal patency, often with apparently normal fimbria, but with distention of the tube proximal to the constricting band. Bands are probably best treated by a single antimesenteric incision in the tube, extending from the distal end through the stenosed segment and through the band. This procedure requires some method of hemostasis. A further consideration is whether this procedure will improve fertility or reduce it because of subsequent adhesion development.

In the patient desirous of conception who has undergone tubal surgery, reassessment of tubal patency should be performed approximately 6–12 weeks postoperatively in most cases. Such follow-up will allow the patient to know whether reocclusion has occurred and thus plan accordingly for assisted-reproduction technology, adoption or to cease in their efforts to conceive.

Tubal anastomosis

Among the various surgical procedures for infertility, the greatest success has probably been achieved with tubal anastomosis: a 70–80% success rate has been seen in women who have undergone prior sterilization procedures; and a 50% success rate in women with pathological obstruction. Factors that influence success include the amount of tube remaining after anastomosis, with an optimal length being at least 4 cm. Coexisting pelvic pathology reduces the likelihood of success as does a disparity between the size of lumina being anastomosed. Another frequently quoted indicator of a poor prognosis is a long duration of time between the tubal ligation and the planned anastomosis. However, this may be more related to the resultant increased age of the patient (which reduces fecundity) rather than the time interval *per se*.

To minimize the morbidity of this procedure, some surgeons have advocated anastomosis at the time of minilaparotomy or endoscopy. It has now been clearly established that either is feasible, although the long-term pregnancy rates with these approaches have yet to be ascertained.

12 Tubal ligation

Tubal ligation should be considered only for women who desire permanent sterilization. Although tubal anastomosis remains an option after tubal ligation, patients should not consent to tubal ligation with the idea that the procedure is readily reversible. On the other hand, patients should also be made aware that the ligation procedure can fail, leading to the possibility of an intrauterine or ectopic pregnancy. The risk of failure of tubal ligation is highly dependent on the technique employed; failure rates are now quoted to be as frequent as approximately one in every 100 operations performed.

Techniques available for tubal ligation include unipolar electrosurgery, bipolar electrosurgery, Fallope rings and Filshie clips (Figure 12.1). Some of these can be performed using a single-puncture approach at the umbilicus to allow the passage of electrosurgical instruments or occluding-device applicators through the operating channel of the laparoscope. Alternatively, the electrosurgical instruments and applicators can be passed through a second-puncture trocar sleeve.

The properties of unipolar and bipolar electrosurgery are different, with greater tissue destruction tending to occur with unipolar procedures (see Figure 3.2). The procedure is usually performed by grasping the tube along the isthmus away from the cornua and coagulating the tissue at three successive sites, progressing from distal to

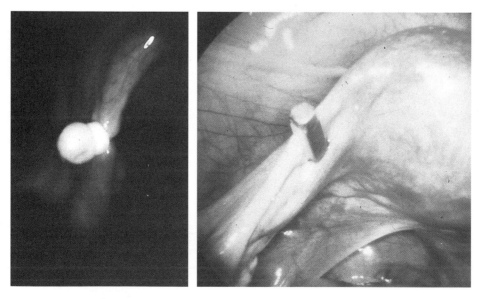

Figure 12.1 Fallope ring *in situ* (left) and a Filshie clip applied to the tube (right) (courtesy of N.D. Motashaw)

proximal. All sites of coagulation should be in the isthmus and not impinge on the cornua. Prior to activation of the electro-surgical generator, care must be taken to ensure that the region is not adherent to adjacent structures. A similar approach is used during bipolar coagulation; the amper-age is monitored and coagulation continued until all flow is stopped at each site. With both procedures, it is important to ensure that the entire diameter of the tube is within the 'paddles' of the electrosurgical grasping instrument. In addition, all of the parts, from electrosurgical generator and the cord from the generator to the endoscope and the grasping instrument itself, should be of the same system model to ensure compatibility and to facilitate the achievement of appropri-ate tissue effects.

When using the mechanical forms of tubal occlusion (such as the Fallope ring or Hulka clip), the tube is also grasped in the isthmic region away from the cornua and then gently elevated before application of the ring / clip, taking care that the entire diameter of the tube is included. Care must be also taken to avoid tearing the tube during this procedure.

A not uncommon cause of failure of tubal ligation is when the procedure is performed on a patient who is already pregnant, often from an earlier phase of the same cycle as during the operation. For this reason, many physicians employ options to minimize such a risk, including only per-forming the procedure when the patient is in the follicular phase of her cycle, obtaining a pregnancy test on the morning of the procedure, performing a dilation and curet-tage as part of the ligation procedure and / or requiring the use of contraception prior to the operation.

An essential in the performance of tubal ligation, regardless of the method employed, is that the structure operated upon is indeed the tube. Because other abdominal structures, such as the bowel, ureter or round ligament, may be mistaken for the Fallopian tube, each tube should be carefully identified and distinguished from the other structures. This is most easily accomplished by identifying the fimbriated end of the tube, then carefully following the tube back from this end to the isthmus.

13 Ovarian surgery

Ovarian surgical procedures fall into three general categories: treatment of small areas of the cortex; ovarian cystectomy; and oophorectomy. A full description of the indications for these procedures and, in particular, the controversy regarding laparoscopic treatment of potentially malignant neoplasms is beyond the scope of this chapter. The reader is referred to other reference sources. In brief, surgical treatment of small areas of the cortex is performed in patients who have superficial endometriotic implants and to aid the induction of ovulation in women with polycystic ovarian (PCO) syndrome. Spots of endometriosis can be treated by a number of modalities, including any of the types of lasers as well as electrosurgery. The goal of such treatment is vaporization / coagulation / ablation of the lesions.

'Ovarian drilling' is one of the terms used to describe the procedure wherein multiple holes are made in the ovarian cortex. These fenestrations allow the follicular fluid, which is rich in androgens, to drain from the ovaries, resulting in a reduction in circulating androgen levels which, in turn, often leads to a concomitant initiation of ovulation. Thus, a 'pseudoovarian wedge resection' is performed. However, this 'correction' of the anovulatory state is often transient and frequently followed by development of periovarian adhesions. Although temporarily facilitating ovulation, the procedure may in fact induce a mechanical cause of infertility.

Ovarian drilling (Figure 13.1) can be carried out by any of a number of modalities,

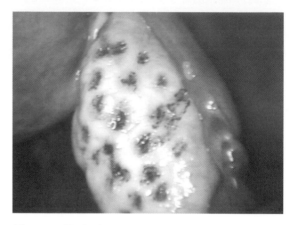

Figure 13.1 Ovarian drilling allows cyst fluid to drain from the ovaries, thereby reducing circulating androgen levels and allowing ovulation (courtesy of D.A. Johns)

including lasers and electrosurgery. The multiple small (approximately 8–12 mm) holes in the ovarian cortex are made over the cysts of similar size often seen circumferentially on the ovaries of women with PCO. Care should be taken not to penetrate too deeply into the ovary towards the hilum of the ovary, as might occur with the use of fiber lasers or unipolar needles, because of the possibility of coagulation of the hilar vessels which will induce a menopausal state.

If the decision is made to perform a procedure endoscopically, then laparoscopic ovarian cystectomy is performed similarly to the approach at laparotomy. An incision is made over the cyst, taking care to avoid perforation of the cyst. The cortex is then grasped and elevated while the wall of the cyst is dissected from its capsule, using a

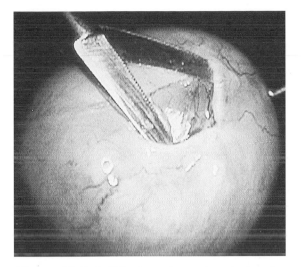

Figure 13.2 A CO_2 laser is used to incise the ovarian cortex, and scissors are used to separate the cyst from the cortex (courtesy of H. Reich)

combination of blunt and sharp dissection (Figure 13.2). On occasions, this process may be facilitated by making several incisions in the surrounding cortex to 'relax' the tissue and to provide sites for grasping the tissue to be excised. Once excised, the cyst is removed either through a posterior colpotomy incision or by placing it in a bag introduced through a trocar sleeve. Once contained within the bag, the cyst is decompressed to allow its extrusion through the trocar sleeve, thereby minimizing contamination of the peritoneal cavity.

Laparoscopic oophorectomy involves isolation of the ovarian vessels in the infundibulopelvic and uteroovarian ligaments. This can be accomplished by electrosurgery, surgical clips or sutures. Regardless of technique, care must be taken to identify the ureter to minimize its risk of injury. Identification of the vessels is facil-itated by dissection of the surrounding tissue to isolate the vessels. Tissue removal is then conducted as during ovarian cystectomy.

As already mentioned in Chapter 10, it may be difficult (if not impossible) to differentiate between a hemorrhagic corpus luteum and an endometrioma at the time of surgery. Thus, the surgeon may occasionally be faced with the dilemma of whether to treat such cysts. Dermoid cysts can often be suspected on the basis of diagnostic imaging studies. An attempt should be made to remove these cysts intact because of the peritonitis that has been described after dermoid rupture. If a dermoid cyst is breached, the sebaceous material should be removed as completely as possible, followed by copious pelvic irrigation.

14 Laparoscopically assisted vaginal hysterectomy

Laparoscopically assisted vaginal hysterectomy (LAVH) is a complex procedure requiring a high level of skill and expertise; it is definitely not a procedure to be attempted by beginners! This procedure has been associated with many complications involving the ureter, bladder, blood vessels and bowel, most of which are likely to be significantly underreported in the literature. Furthermore, even among those procedures that are successfully completed, many are of a marathon duration or require blood transfusions that are likely to have placed the patient at greater risk than if the procedure had been performed vaginally or abdominally.

The controversy surrounding LAVH is compounded by a lack of a clear-cut definition of what the procedure is. There has been a recent attempt to establish a classification system for LAVH to allow comparison with equivalent alternative therapeutic options (Table 14.1). The proposed system is based on the part of the procedure that is performed laparoscopically.

LAVH should be a means of converting what would have been an abdominal hysterectomy into a vaginal hysterectomy, which is associated with a lower rate of morbidity compared with the abdominal approach. However, the outcome of LAVH is highly variable because of the diverse levels of expertise and experience of surgeons with open, vaginal and laparoscopic approaches. Thus, the relative contraindications for LAVH will vary among surgeons (Table 14.2).

Of the many approaches available for carrying out LAVH, only one is described here, although others are equally satisfactory. This approach includes complete extirpation

Table 14.1 Classification of laparoscopically assisted vaginal hysterectomy (LAVH)

Stage	Description
0	Laparoscopy carried out with no laparoscopic procedure performed prior to vaginal hysterectomy
1	Procedure includes laparoscopic adhesiolysis and / or excision of endometriosis
2	Either or both adnexa are laparoscopically freed
3	Bladder laparoscopically dissected from uterus
4	Uterine artery laparoscopically transected
5	Anterior and / or posterior colpotomy or entire uterus laparoscopically freed
Subscript	
0	Neither ovary excised
1	One ovary excised
2	Both ovaries excised

NB: If the extent of the laparoscopic procedure differed between the right and left pelvic side walls, the procedure is staged according to the most advanced side

Reproduced from Johns and Diamond, *J Reprod Med* 1994;39:424–8, with permission

Table 14.2 Relative clinical contraindications for LAVH

Enlarged uterus

Prior Cesarean section

Prior pelvic surgery

Presence of pelvic pain

Known pelvic adhesions

Ectopic pregnancy

Presence of endometriosis

History of pelvic inflammatory disease

Undiagnosed pelvic mass

Bowel or appendix disorder

Nulliparity

Prior uterus suspension

Lack of uterine descensus

Uterine or cervical cancer

Planned bilateral salpingo-oophorectomy

of the uterus, tubes and ovaries laparoscopically, although this can be converted to a vaginal procedure at any stage, according to the preferences of the surgeon.

The procedure is initiated using a three-puncture approach to accommodate the laparoscope at the umbilicus and lower bilateral secondary trocars. An instrument can be placed transvaginally in the uterus to facilitate manipulation. After determining the location of the ureter, the round ligament is grasped with a bipolar electrosurgical instrument and coagulated, then cut with a peritoneal incision that extends both over the anterior uterine surface and back towards the infundibulopelvic ligament. (If the plan is to spare the tubes and ovaries, then the incision is directed towards the uteroovarian ligament, which is grasped, coagulated and incised.) Using blunt dissection or aqua dissection (wherein irrigating solution is sprayed under high pressure along the intended plane of dissection to separate the tissues), the infundibulopelvic ligaments can be separated from the side walls of the pelvis and the ureters identified bilaterally.

The peritoneal incisions can then be joined in the midline overlying the uterus.

After freeing the infundibulopelvic ligaments, the underlying peritoneum can then be opened either through the space created by the dissection or through the pelvic side wall. The peritoneum over the infundibulopelvic vessels is incised, and the vessels occluded by electrosurgery, clips and / or suture ties and transected. The same procedure is followed on the contralateral side. At this stage, the uterus can be retroverted to facilitate dissection of the bladder away from the lower uterine segment. Using a uterine manipulator, the uterus can then be deviated away from the broad ligament to be incised by a combination of electrosurgery and sharp dissection, bearing in mind the location of the ureter to avoid its inadvertent transection. This incision is carried on to the level of the uterine vessels bilaterally; the peritoneum over the posterior aspect of the cervix between the uterosacral ligaments is then incised. The isolated uterine vessels can then be occluded using electrosurgery, clips (Figure 14.1), suture or other method. The uterosacral ligaments are incised bilaterally, followed by incision of the cardinal ligaments.

The vagina is entered and the incision extended circumferentially around the cervix to completely extirpate the uterus, tubes and ovaries, which are removed vaginally. The vaginal cuff is closed either vaginally or laparoscopically, using sutures in a figure-eight pattern, beginning at the cardinal ligaments to provide support of the vaginal angles. The uterosacral ligaments are incorporated into the closure to further support the vagina.

On completion of closure, the surgical site is laparoscopically inspected to assess hemostasis. (Such an inspection is also an option for procedures completed vaginally. If the laparoscope is left in place when the

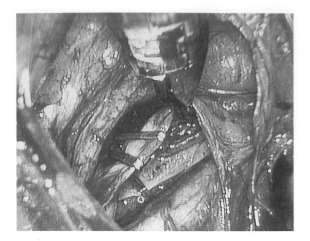

Figure 14.1 Two clips have been put on the uterine artery and, in this case, on the vein (below) as well. A fourth clip may be placed on the uterine side to prevent backflow during further surgery (courtesy of J. Deprest)

procedure is converted to a vaginal approach, the abdomen can be reinsufflated after vaginal closure and the vaginal cuff inspected for bleeding sites.) At this stage, the laparoscopic instruments and trocar sleeves can be removed as described in Chapter 6.

Recently, endoscopic approaches have also been employed to treat pelvic malignancies. Such procedures include radical hysterectomy, pelvic and para-aortic lymphadenectomy, and staging and second-look procedures for ovarian cancer. Individual surgery can be successful with these procedures although, as yet, there remains only limited long-term follow-up of patients who have undergone such surgery and limited acceptance of the adequacy of such dissections. Similarly, surgeons have clearly demonstrated the feasibility of bowel resection and anastomosis, large and small bowel repair, and genitourinary repairs. However, it is my opinion that the treatment of these complications should be performed only by advanced endoscopic surgeons who consider themselves competent to perform such procedures at laparotomy. In addition, it is also my opinion that a complication (such as an unintentional bowel injury) is best treated by conventional approaches, with the liberal involvement of consultants (if readily available). However, it should be recognized that conventional approaches will vary from surgeon to surgeon according to their specific experience, training and expertise.

15 Laparoscopic treatment of stress incontinence and other pelvic floor defects

C.H. Nezhat, F.R. Nezhat and C.R. Nezhat

Introduction

By the year 2000, 20% of the population will be over 65 years of age, and 50% of women aged 50 years today will live into their tenth decade. 'Baby-boomers' are approaching menopause and do not want to live with the associated problems of aging such as urogenital prolapse and stress urinary incontinence (SUI). In fact, not only do baby-boomers want treatment for themselves, but they encourage their elders (mothers and grandmothers) to seek treatment as well. Urine leakage, genital protrusion and the associated inconveniences are not an acceptable outcome of being female; these women have abandoned the 'born-to-live-with-it' school of thought.

Bothersome protrusion and pelvic pressure that worsen with ambulation and daily activity are common presenting symptoms. Other symptoms include difficulty in walking, urinary incontinence, difficulty in voiding or defecating, recurrent mucosal irritation, ulceration, coital difficulty and problems with hygiene. However, the protruding mass that limits activity and social outings is the overriding complaint of the condition. A variety of operations, including both vaginal and abdominal approaches, has been described for treatment of pelvic support defects.

Preoperative evaluation

A detailed examiniation and knowledge of pelvic anatomy are essential components of the approach to reconstructive pelvic surgery. All anatomical defects are identified and the operation is planned with the intention to correct each defect to maximize optimal outcome[1,2]. In addition, the patient who is a candidate for laparoscopy should be able to tolerate general anesthesia, increased intra-abdominal pressure and Trendelenburg positioning. Appropriate bowel preparation instructions are given as indicated[3].

Laparoscopic technique

Emphasizing the principles of the trans-abdominal approach, laparoscopy has evolved as an alternative technique in reconstructive pelvic surgery while maintaining sexual function capacity[1,2]. The advantages of laparoscopy over laparotomy include a smaller incision, elimination of abdominal packing, less manipulation of the viscera, a better view of the pelvis and precise hemostasis.

Laparoscopic reconstructive pelvic surgery is mainly performed under general anesthesia following the same principles of technique as in laparotomy. The patient receives a dose of intravenous antibiotics prophylactically. After induction of general endotracheal anesthesia, a 10–11-mm umbilical trocar and three lower-abdominal 5-mm ancillary trocars (two lateral to the epigastric vessels at the level of the iliac crest and one in the midline 5 cm above the pubic symphysis; Figure 15.1) are placed. The patient is then placed in the Trendelenburg position and

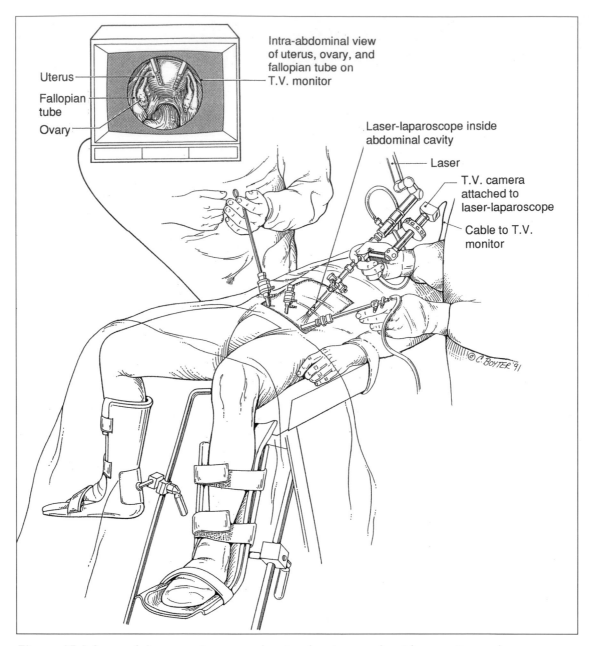

Figure 15.1 Setup of the operating room showing the view on the video monitor and the location of the suprapubic incisions

tilted to the left to shift the bowel away from the operating field. After a thorough evaluation of the peritoneal cavity and completion of other procedures such as hysterectomy, lysis of adhesions or removal of the adnexa, pelvic reconstruction can proceed.

Bladder-neck suspension

Urinary incontinence is becoming more prevalent as the population ages[4,5], with as much as 20–40% of women reporting urine loss[4–7]. This disorder has a profound effect on the individual as well as on the general population. The psychological status of these patients improves significantly after successful surgical cure of genuine SUI[8]. However, with more than 160 corrective operations available, an optimal approach has yet to be determined[9].

Among the available procedures, retropubic urethropexy, and both Marshall–Marchetti–Krantz[10] and Burch[11,12], produce the best outcomes with relatively few complications. Needle urethropexy[13–17] is associated with shorter operating times and recovery periods, and is less invasive. However, it is less effective than the abdominal approach, and is associated with more complications[18–21]. Tanagho's modification of the Burch procedure[22] is reported to have the best outcome in patients with pure genuine SUI and intact urethral sphincteric mechanism[22–26]. Laparoscopic bladder-neck suspension has been performed with good results[27–30].

Laparoscopic retropubic urethral suspension combines an outpatient procedure with a potentially longterm solution to SUI. Advantages include excellent retropubic exposure and access due to videolaparoscopic magnification, which enhances the surgeon's ability to place sutures precisely. In addition, the improved exposure allows support restoration with limited mobility and avoids urethral obstruction and compression. Patients receive the social and financial advantages of a short recovery, including an early return to the workplace. Laparoscopic retropubic colposuspension using the Burch method has been associated with the best outcome and relatively few complications[30].

Preoperative evaluation should include history and physical, gynecological and neurological examinations. Attempts should be made to evaluate and correct, if possible, any factor contributing to urinary incontinence, for example, drugs or respiratory disease. Office tests include stress tests (lithotomy and standing), the Q-Tip® test, urinalysis, urine culture and sensitivity, and blood chemistry. Also recommended is a multichannel urodynamic evaluation in the lithotomy and standing positions with emphasis on voiding time, voiding volume and postvoid residual urine volume. Tests include a waterfill cystometrogram with continuous urethral pressure monitoring, and subtracted rectal and abdominal pressures. Genuine SUI is diagnosed by a positive stress test in the absence of simultaneous detrusor contractions or pressure equalization on the stress urethral closure-pressure profile. Patients are encouraged to keep 24–48-h symptom diaries.

Operative technique

After induction of general endotracheal anesthesia, the patient is placed in Allen stirrups, which permit the assistant to perform a vaginal examination. A Foley catheter is placed in the urethra and bladder. A 10-mm operative videolaparoscope is inserted infraumbilically, and three 5-mm accessory cannulas are inserted. The middle cannula is 5–6 cm above the pubic symphysis, and the other two are 7–8 cm above the pubic symphysis and lateral to the epigastric vessels. A carbon dioxide (CO_2) laser is placed through the operative channel of the 10-mm laparoscope and used as a long knife. A suction irrigator, grasping forceps, needle holder and bipolar electrocoagulator[3] are introduced through the accessory cannulas.

The intraperitoneal cavity is carefully inspected to detect any pelvic abnormalities requiring surgical treatment such as adhesions or endometriosis. First, any indicated gynecological procedures are performed, for example, hysterectomy with or without removal of adnexa, treatment of endometriosis or adhesions, or enterocele repair. After identifying the ureters, a culdoplasty is performed if indicated. The enterocele sac is excised and a laparoscopic pursestring suture (1-0 polybutilate-coated polyester) is used, beginning at the bottom of the cul-de-sac and exercising care to incorporate the posterior wall of the vagina, only the peritoneum laterally at the left and right pararectal areas, and only shallow bites of serosa over the anterior rectosigmoid colon. In patients who have undergone previous hysterectomy, any remnant of the uterosacral ligaments is included in the suture. Closure of the cul-de-sac should leave no defect that could result in bowel entrapment.

Transperitoneal technique

This is one of the various techniques that can be used to enter the space of Retzius. The anterior abdominal wall peritoneum 5–7 cm above the pubic symphysis is pulled down, using grasping forceps placed through a lateral accessory cannula (Figure 15.2). A transverse incision is made with the CO_2 laser or scissors caudal to the midsuprapubic cannula above the pubic symphysis on the peritoneum between the two umbilical liga-ments. The midline cannula entry and anatomical landmarks, including the round ligament from the internal ring, are used to avoid injury to the bladder. Retropubic space dissection is carried on bluntly with hydrodissection, or with scissors or the CO_2 laser for sharp dissection (Figure 15.3). Care is taken to stay close to the back of the pubic bone, dropping the anterior bladder wall, vaginal wall and urethra downward. Dissection is limited over the urethra in the midline to approximately 2 cm lateral to the urethra to protect its delicate musculature. An assistant performs a vaginal examination with one finger on each side of the catheterized urethra, elevating the lateral vaginal fornix. The overlying fibrofatty tissue is cleared from the anterior vaginal wall under videolaparoscopic magnification. Beginning laterally, the bladder is dissected medially from the paravaginal fascia. The thin-walled venous plexus in this extremely vascularized area is identified and protected from surgical trauma.

Balloon dissection

The balloon dissector (General Surgical Innovations, Inc., Portola Valley, CA) consists

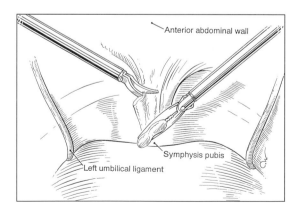

Figure 15.2 An incision is made in the peritoneum 3–5 cm above the pubic symphysis

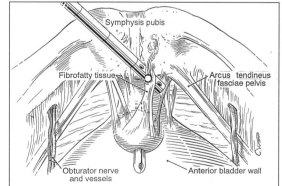

Figure 15.3 The space of Retzius is developed using blunt and CO_2 laser dissection of fibrofatty tissue. Care is taken to avoid injury to the obturator nerve and vessels

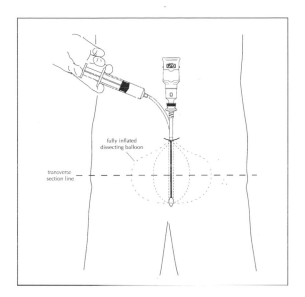

Figure 15.4 The balloon dissector is inserted infraumbilically and advanced to the pubic symphysis. The balloon is shown in partial expansion within the extraperitoneal space

of a cannula, guide rod and balloon system. The dissector is inserted through a 1-cm infraumbilical incision (Figure 15.4), and advanced between the rectus muscle and anterior surface of the posterior rectus sheath to the pubic symphysis. The external sheath of the dissector is then removed and the balloon inflated with approximately 750 mL of saline solution. During inflation, the balloon unrolls sideways and exerts a perpendicular force that separates the tissue layers (Figure 15.5). Blunt dissection of the connective tissues is propagated as the balloon expands. When maximum volume is reached, the balloon is deflated and removed

through the incision. The dissected space is insufflated with CO_2 gas at a pressure of 8–10 mmHg. The predefined shape of the balloon, its non-elastomeric material and the incompressible nature of the saline ensure a large, relatively bloodless, working space of a predictable size and shape. The space is adequate for identifying pertinent landmarks and for unencumbered manipulation of endoscopic surgical instruments.

Preperitoneal technique

This method of accessing the space of Retzius employs the same patient position and trocar placement as described above. To begin dissection of the space, a midsuprapubic cannula is inserted into the preperitoneal area and a 16-gauge laparoscopic needle is introduced through it. Approximately 30–50 mL of dilute vasopressin (20 units in 60–100 mL of Ringer's lactate solution) is injected subperitoneally in the lower anterior abdominal wall above the bladder to decrease oozing. The needle is replaced by a suction irrigator probe, and 300–500 mL of Ringer's lactate solution or normal saline is injected at a pressure of 300 mmHg to form a subperitoneal space in the anterior abdominal wall.

The videolaparoscope is retracted from the abdominal cavity and directed towards the newly created subperitoneal space. A long hydrodissection probe is inserted through the space under direct observation and the space further expanded, using

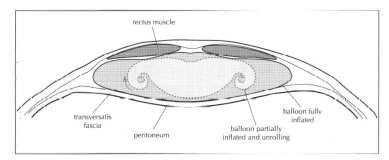

Figure 15.5 Seen in the transverse plane, as the balloon is inflated with saline solution, it unrolls and dissects the tissue layers

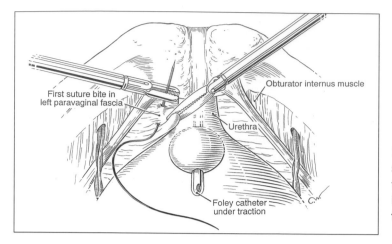

First suture bite in
left paravaginal fascia

Obturator internus muscle

Urethra

Foley catheter
under traction

Figure 15.6 An 0 Ethibond suture is placed 1–1.5 cm from the urethra. The assistant's finger is used to elevate the paravaginal fascia and guide the surgeon

hydrodissection. The videolaparoscope is advanced into this space, which is insufflated with CO_2 gas. The lateral suprapubic trocars are retracted to the pneumosubperitoneal space. Blunt or, on occasions, sharp dissection may be required to lyse adhesions that remain following hydrodissection. At this point, the pubic symphysis and Cooper's ligaments can be seen. The patient may be placed in the deep Trendelenburg position and rotated to the left to facilitate left-handed suture placement.

Our experience with the first 10 cases using this technique has been reported[31], and resulted in good outcomes with no complications. The technique has several advantages over transperitoneal and balloon dissection[3,30]. Extension of the peritoneal incision is avoided, eliminating repair and minimizing the risks of bowel herniation and adhesion formation. The danger of surgical trauma to the thin-walled venous plexus in this well-vascularized area during blunt or sharp dissection is minimized.

Although the balloon dissector is an effective alternative to manual dissection of the space of Retzius[30], it is more costly to use. Furthermore, the balloon, which should be inserted between the rectus muscle and anterior surface of the posterior rectus sheath, may be inadvertently advanced into

an incorrect plane. The predefined shape of the balloon and its non-elastomeric material may force dissection that is less dependent on patient anatomical planes.

Suspension technique

After dissection of the space of Retzius by any of the above-described routes is complete and the paravaginal fascia is identified, using an atraumatic grasping forceps, a bite of the paravaginal fascia is elevated and a 1-0 polybutilate-coated polyester endoscopic suture on a tapered 2.2 cm straight or curved needle is placed at the level of the urethrovesical junction approximately 1–1.5 cm from the urethra (Figure 15.6). The assistant's finger is used as a guide, facilitated by placing the bulb of a Foley catheter under gentle traction. The suture is placed perpendicular to the vaginal axis to include approximately 1–2 cm of tissue (the complete vaginal fascia), but not the vaginal mucosa, and is fixed to Cooper's ligament (Figure 15.7). The sutures are tied intra- or extracorporeally with the help of an assistant, who lifts the vagina upwards and forwards (Figure 15.8). Direct visualization allows the surgeon to gauge the tension in the vaginal wall while tying the sutures. The urethra is observed to ensure that it is not

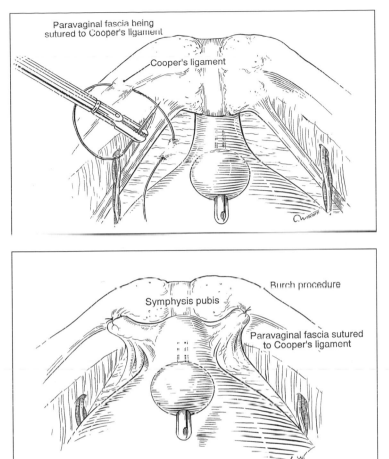

Figure 15.7 The suture is passed through Cooper's ligament in the Burch procedure

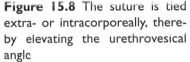

Figure 15.8 The suture is tied extra- or intracorporeally, thereby elevating the urethrovesical angle

compressed against the pubic bone. Suturing is repeated on the opposite side to create a platform on which the bladder neck can rest while avoiding cinching. If the suspension is judged inadequate by visual inspection, manual elevation or cystoscopy, a second set of sutures may be placed cephalad along the base of the bladder.

Cystoscopy is performed to ensure that there is no suture material in the bladder, and to assess the angle of the urethrovesical junction and urethral patency. Pneumosubperitoneal pressure is decreased and the retropubic space is thoroughly evaluated. Bleeding is controlled with the bipolar electrocoagulator. The laparoscope is then withdrawn from the space of Retzius into

the abdomen. No drain is used and the peritoneal defect is closed with an absorbable suture. The laparoscope is removed from the abdomen and the procedure completed. The transurethral Foley catheter is left in place for 2–3 days, and all patients need to be instructed on self-catheterization. Patients should receive perioperative first-generation cephalosporin as intravenous antibiotic prophylaxis, followed by a course of oral antibiotics for 5 days or until self catheterization is discontinued, whichever is the longer.

In our first series of 62 women, one bladder perforation occurred during bladder dissection and entry into the space of Retzius. It was repaired laparoscopically in one layer, using 0 polyglactin interrupted sutures. One patient, who had oophorectomy also, developed an incisional hernia at the site of the midline suprapubic cannula, although the fascia had been repaired with one interrupted absorbable suture. The repair was carried out as an outpatient with good results. Another patient was unable to void postoperatively and required self-catheterization for 10 days. Nine women had dysuria without infection that resolved with phenazopyridine hydrochloride (Pyridium™) treatment.

During the 8–30-month follow-up, all patients reported satisfactory relief of symptoms with subjective and objective improvement. None experienced urinary leakage during activities similar to those preoperatively associated with their condition. Subjective success was determined by a questionnaire on urinary leakage, and the absence of a need to wear pads (none were required). Objective success was assessed by comparison of pre- and postoperative symptom diaries, urine characteristics by straight-catheter postvoid residual volume, urethrovesical junction angle as determined by catheter and / or Q-Tip placement, bladder support and negative standing stress test[30].

Paravaginal repair

Vaginal reconstructive surgery for pelvic organ prolapse is one of the most challenging aspects of surgical gynecology, and recurrence is particularly troublesome in the anterior vagina. Cystocele and its companion urethrocele have been described as herniations or defects in the bladder and urethra, respectively.

Paravaginal repair is required when cystourethrocele is the result of a separation of the pubocervical fascia from its lateral attachment to the pelvic sidewall. When this defect is accompanied by genuine SUI, the carefully performed paravaginal repair will almost always correct the SUI[32].

Paravaginal repair is simply an attempt to restore normal anatomy. Dissection during anterior colporrhaphy splits the vaginal muscularis, and repair involves plication of the muscularis and adventitia (not vaginal 'fascia') in the midline, which may pull the lateral attachments further from the pelvic sidewall. Paravaginal repair restores the lateral attachments to the pelvic sidewall at the linea alba. Reported failure rates range from 0–20% with anterior colporrhaphy and 3–14% with paravaginal repair[33].

Four different pubocervical fascial defects can cause cystocele: the paravaginal defect; transverse defect; midline defect; and distal defect. Distinguishing the various defects is particularly important as each type of defect requires a different procedure. Differentiation requires a knowledge of normal anatomy and careful observation.

The paravaginal defect is a result of detachment of the pubocervical fascia from its lateral attachment to the fascia of the internal obturator muscle at the level of the arcus tendineus fascia of the pelvis[34–36]. This is the most common cause of cystourethrocele. The repair consists of reestablishing the lateral pelvic sidewall attachments of the pubocervical fascia and restoring stability of this 'hammock' by correcting the fundamental anatomical defect in this type of cystourethrocele.

The transverse defect is due to transverse separation of the pubocervical fascia from the pericervical ring into which the cardinal and uterosacral ligaments insert. The base of the bladder herniates into the anterior vaginal fornix and forms a pure cystocele without displacing the urethra or urethrovesical junction.

The midline or central defect is caused by a break in the central portion of the hammock between its lateral, dorsal or ventral attachments.

The distal defect is rare, but it does occur. The distal urethra becomes avulsed or separated from its attachment to the urogenital diaphragm as it passes under the pubic symphysis.

Operative technique

The retropubic space is entered and dissected as described above. Anatomical landmarks such as the pubic symphysis, obturator foramen and obturator neurovascular bundle are identified. The paravaginal defect (lateral vaginal sulci) can be seen detaching from the arcus tendineus fascia of the pelvis.

The bladder is mobilized medially and the pubocervical fascia exposed. The ischial spine is located digitally by the operator's fingers inside the vagina while viewing through the laparoscope. During mobilization of the bladder, the lateral superior sulcus of the vagina is lifted by the assistant's fingers in the vagina to facilitate dissection.

Separation of the lateral sulcus from the pelvic sidewall can easily be appreciated laparoscopically. Permanent sutures such as 2-0 prolene are used to suture the superior lateral sulcus of the vagina to the arcus tendineus fascia of the pelvis (linea alba). The superior lateral sulcus of the vagina is elevated by the assistant's fingers in the vagina, going beneath the prominent paraurethral vascular plexus if possible, and sutured to the linea alba of the pelvic sidewall.

The paraurethral vascular plexus, which runs longitudinally along the axis of the vagina, can be identified on magnification through the videolaparoscope and electrodessicated prior to suture placement. Otherwise, bleeding may occur when the plexus is penetrated by the needle. Such bleeding invariably stops when the suspension sutures are tied. To avoid bleeding contamination of the operative field, the first paravaginal suspension stitch should be placed as close to the ischial spine as possible. Figure-of-eight sutures are used on all suspension stitches to obtain better hemostasis and suspension. Following placement of the first stitch, additional sutures are placed through the vaginal sulcus with its overlying fascia and the arcus tendineus fascia lying ventrally toward the pubic symphysis. The last stitch should be as close as possible to the pubic ramus ventrally.

It is important not to injure the pudendal vessels and nerve when making the first stitch. Before placing the first stitch, the surgeon should clearly identify the ischial spine by vaginal palpation and viewing through the laparoscope. The first stitch is usually placed through the linea alba approximately 1–1.5 cm ventral to the ischial spine[37]. Frequent vaginal examination is performed while suturing to aid proper placement, and to assess the adequacy of suspension and reestablishment of the anterior support. The procedure is completed by bladder-neck suspension as described above.

Vaginal vault suspension (sacral colpopexy)

Vaginal vault prolapse occurs when the apex of the vagina descends below the introitus, turning the vagina inside-out. It is uncommon in the USA, affecting only 900–1200 women annually[38].

The different approaches to treatment of vaginal vault prolapse include the use of a pessary (non-surgical), vaginal reconstruction (functional) and vaginal closure (obliterative). For the latter, patient selection criteria include physiological age, sexual interest or desire, general health status and symptomatology.

More and more women now remain sexually active and wish to preserve coital capacity. In such cases, total colpocleisis is not an option, leaving reconstruction and suspension of the vaginal vault. The goal of this procedure is to correct all anatomical defects, maintain or restore normal bowel and bladder function, and retain the vaginal canal for sexual function. Transvaginal sacrospinous vault suspension and needle urethropexy have shown as much as a 67% optimal or satisfactory outcome[39].

Thus, the vaginal route may certainly be used in women whose preference or medical disorders contraindicate the abdominal approach. However, studies have shown a 33% rate of recurrent prolapse associated with sacrospinous fixation and transvaginal needle suspension[39]. The abdominal approach has been found to be more effective than the vaginal route in treating urogenital prolapse. The probability for optimal surgical outcome is twice as great with a transabdominal operation, and the chances of an unsatisfactory surgical outcome by transvaginal repair are twice as great.

Among the proposed surgical techniques to prevent and correct this condition is abdominal sacral colpopexy, comprising the interposition of a synthetic suspensory hammock between the prolapsed vaginal vault and anterior surface of the sacrum[40–42]. However, this technique usually requires a midline abdominal incision, abdominal packing and extensive bowel manipulation, and has a potential for morbidity such as infection, wound separation or dehiscence, and ileus or bowel obstruction[42]. To minimize these drawbacks, we have modified sacral colpopexy to be performed laparoscopically.

Patient evaluation and preparation for surgery should focus on the degree of prolapse and associated rectocele, cystourethrocele and incontinence (urinary or fecal). Instructions for a preoperative mechanical and antibiotic bowel preparation are given.

Operative technique

After the induction of general endotracheal anesthesia, and introduction of the operative laparoscope and ancillary 5-mm suprapubic trocars as described above, the patient is placed in the Trendelenburg position and tilted to the left to move the bowel away from the operating field. After a thorough evaluation of the peritoneal cavity and completion of other procedures, such as hysterectomy or lysis of adhesions, the vaginal vault is elevated by a sponge on a ring forceps. The vaginal apex is prepared by removing peritoneum and connective tissue until the vaginal fascia and scar are seen (Figure 15.9). The bladder

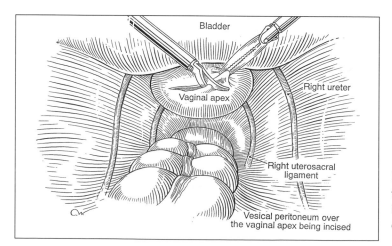

Figure 15.9 The vesicle peritoneum over the vaginal apex is incised, and the vaginal apex is cleaned

is dissected from the anterior vaginal wall and the rectum from the posterior vaginal wall so that approximately 4 cm of the vaginal vault is exposed. If the vagina is opened in cases of hysterectomy or partial vaginectomy, pneumoperitoneum is maintained by placing an inflated surgical glove in the vagina (Ceana's glove).

Repair of an enterocele is performed laparoscopically by excising the sac and using a modified Moschcowitz procedure as described above. The rectosigmoid colon is pushed to the left to expose the sacral area. The posterior parietal peritoneum at or below the sacral promontory is lifted with grasping forceps and incised to the level of the third and fourth sacral vertebrae (S3–S4), and the anterior sacral fascia is exposed. The peritoneal incision is extended from the right pararectal area downwards towards the vagina through the presacral space (Figure 15.10). The following anatom-

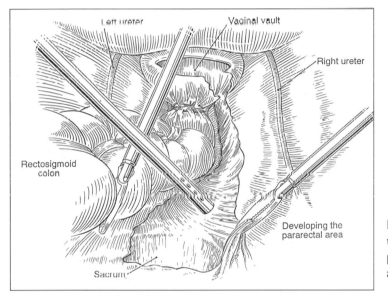

Figure 15.10 Using hydrodissection and the CO_2 laser, the right pararectal and presacral spaces are developed

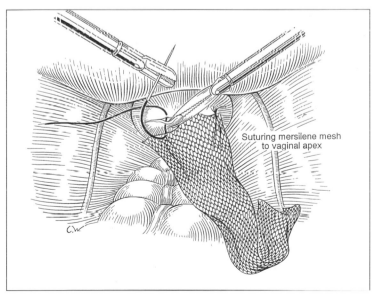

Figure 15.11 The mersilene mesh is tied very loosely to the vaginal apex

ical landmarks are identified: right ureter; internal iliac artery and vein; descending colon; and presacral vessels.

A 2.5×10-cm piece of mersilene or Gore-Tex™ (W.L. Gore and Associates, Inc., Phoenix, AZ) mesh is rolled and introduced into the abdomen through the 10-mm suprapubic or umbilical port. Three to five 0 Ethibond sutures (Ethicon, Inc., Somerville, NJ) are placed in a single row in the posterior vaginal wall apex (excluding the vaginal mucosa) from one lateral fornix to the other. Each suture is placed through one end of the mesh and loosely tied (Figure 15.11).

Other supportive measures in the lower vagina, such as anterior and posterior colpor-

rhaphy, may be necessary for the lower and middle third of the vagina. If required, partial vaginectomy is accomplished. The mesh is sutured to the posterior vaginal wall with non-absorbable suture and placed intraperitoneally before closing the vaginal cuff with delayed-absorbable sutures.

The mesh is adjusted to hold the vaginal apex in the correct anatomical postion without being tight. Two permanent sutures or staples are placed in the longitudinal ligaments of the anterior surface of the sacrum approximately 1-cm apart, in the midline over S3–S4 (Figure 15.12). The peritoneum is then sutured over the graft from the sacrum towards the vagina. Usually,

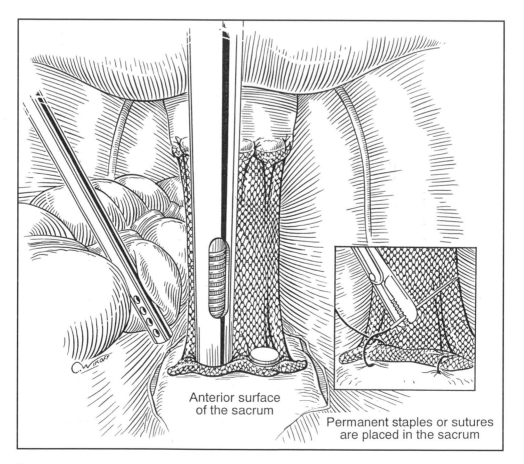

Anterior surface
of the sacrum

Permanent staples or sutures
are placed in the sacrum

Figure 15.12 Two permanent sutures or staples are placed in the presacral ligament approximately 1-cm apart in the midline over the S3–S4 vertebrae

only a small segment of the graft cannot be covered. The serosa of the tail of the bladder (posterior peritoneal fold) and the superficial serosa of the sigmoid colon are used to cover the exposed mesh completely (Figure 15.13). If indicated, laparoscopic urethropexy is performed at this point.

Postoperatively, the patient is given instructions to limit her activity, and to avoid intercourse for 6 weeks, and strenuous exercise and heavy lifting for 2 months. Diet is advanced as tolerated, and a mild laxative prescribed to prevent constipation.

In our first reported series of 15 women, one patient had substantial bleeding during the application of presacral staples to anchor the mesh to the sacrum that required laparotomy. The patients were followed for 3–40 months; all indicated complete relief of their symptoms, with excellent vaginal vault support and no coital difficulty[43].

Conclusions

Although the principles of an abdominal approach are followed, the disadvantages of a laparotomy incision are avoided. Because the sutures are deep in the pelvis, the problems with bolsters and sutures that occur with needle procedures are unusual with laparoscopy. Elevation of the bladder neck depends on the scarring of the para-

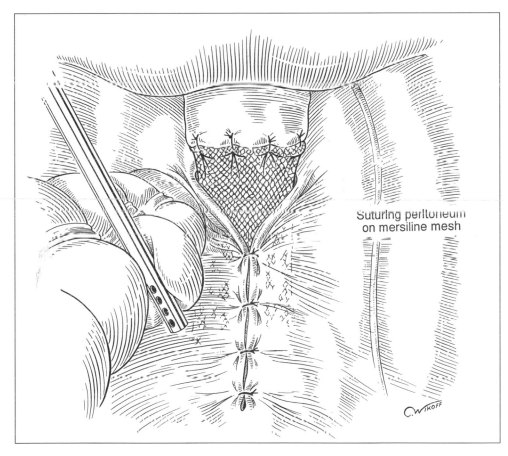

Suturing peritoneum on mersiline mesh

Figure 15.13 Sutures or staples can be used to retroperitonealize the mesh

vesical tissue to the pubic symphysis or pelvic sidewall, not on the two paraurethral sutures as in the needle procedure. Furthermore, this is not a blind operation, and we consider the visualization to be better than at laparotomy.

Unlike transvaginally, laparoscopy allows diagnosis and prompt treatment of pelvic pathology such as endometriosis and

adhesions, and the removal of diseased organs if necessary. We believe that genuine SUI may be corrected laparoscopically with comparable results to laparotomy[27–30], and we have found such an operation to be less traumatic and invasive, with decreases in operative and postoperative recovery times, and in morbidity.

References

1. Nichols DH, Randall CL, eds. *Vaginal Surgery*, 4th edn. Baltimore: Williams & Wilkins, 1996

2. Thompson JD, Rock JA, eds. *Te Linde's Operative Gynecology*, 7th edn. Philadelphia: J.B. Lippincott, 1992

3. Nezhat C, Nezhat F, Luciano A, *et al. Operative Gynecologic Laparoscopy: Principles and Techniques*. New York: McGraw–Hill, 1995

4. Thomas TM, Plymat DR, Blannin J, *et al.* Prevalence of urinary incontinence. *Br Med J* 1980;281:1243–5

5. Diokno AC, Brock BM, Brown MD, *et al.* Prevalence of urinary incontinence and other urological symptoms in the non-institutionalized elderly. *J Urol* 1986;136:1022–5

6. Yarnell JW, St Leger AS. The prevalence, severity and factors associated with urinary incontinence in a random sample of the elderly. *Age Aging* 1979;8:81–5

7. Holst K, Wilson PD. The prevalence of female urinary incontinence and reasons for not seeking treatment. *NZ Med J* 1988;101:756–8

8. Rosenzweig BA, Hischke MD, Thomas S, *et al.* Stress incontinence in women: Psychological status before and after treatment. *J Reprod Med* 1991;36:835–8

9. Horbach NS. Genuine SUI: Best surgical approach. *Comtemp OB/GYN* 1992; 37:53–61

10. Marshall VF, Marchetti AA, Krantz KE. The correction of stress incontinence by simple vesicourethral suspension. *Surg Gynecol Obstet* 1941;88:509–18

11. Burch JC. Cooper's ligament urethrovesical suspension for stress incontinence. *Am J Obstet Gynecol* 1968;100:764–72

12. Stanton SL. Colposuspension. In Stanton SL, Tanagho E, eds. *Surgery of Female Incontinence*, 2nd edn. New York: Springer-Verlag, 1986: 95–103

13. McGuire EJ, Lytton B. Pubovaginal sling procedure for stress incontinence. *J Urol* 1978;119:82–4

14. Pereyra AJ, Lebherz TB. Combined urethrovesical suspension and vaginourethroplasty for correction of urinary stress incontinence. *Obstet Gynecol* 1967;30:537–46

15. Raz S. Modified bladder neck suspension for female stress incontinence. *Urology* 1981;17: 82–5

16. Hohnfellner R, Petrie E. Sling procedures in surgery. In Stanton SL, Tanagho E, eds. *Surgery of Female Incontinence*, 2nd edn. New York: Springer-Verlag, 1986:105–13

17. Gittes RF, Loughlin KR. No incision pubovaginal suspension for stress incontinence. *J Urol* 1987;138:568–70

18. Bhatia NN, Bergman A. A modified Burch versus Pereyra retropubic urethropexy for stress urinary incontinence. *Obstet Gynecol* 1985;66:255–61

19. Mundy AR. A trial comparing the Stamey bladder neck suspension procedure with colposuspension for the treatment of stress incontinence. *Br J Urol* 1983;33:687–90

20. Green DF, McGuire EJ, Lytton B. A comparison of endoscopic suspension of the vesical neck versus anterior urethropexy for the treatment of stress urinary incontinence. *J Urol* 1986;136:1205–7

21. Karram MM, Bhatia NN. Transvaginal needle bladder neck suspension procedures for stress urinary incontinence: A comprehensive review. *Obstet Gynecol* 1989;73:906–14

22. Tanagho EA. Colpocystourethropexy: The way we do it. *J Urol* 1976;116:751–3

23. Bergman A, Ballard C, Koonings P. Primary stress urinary incontinence and pelvic relaxation: Prospective randomized comparison of three different operations. *Am J Obstet Gynecol* 1989;161:97–101

24. Bergman A, Ballard C, Koonings P. Comparison of three different surgical procedures for genuine stress incontinence: Prospective randomized study. *Am J Obstet Gynecol* 1989;160:1102–6

25. Penttinen J, Kindholm EL, Kaar K, et al. Successful colposuspension in stress urinary incontinence reduces bladder neck mobility and increases pressure transmission to the urethra. *Acta Gynecol Obstet* 1989;224:233–8

26. van Geelen JM, Theeuwes AGM, Eskes IKAB, et al. The clinical and urodynamic effects of anterior vaginal repair and Burch colposuspension. *Am J Obstet Gynecol* 1989; 159:137–44

27. Vancaillie TG, Schuessler W. Laparoscopic bladderneck suspension. *J Laparoendosc Surg* 1991;1:169–73

28. Nezhat CH, Roemisch M, Siedman DS, et al. Laparoscopic colposuspension, a new surgical approach. *Contemp OB/GYN* 1997;41: 70–84

29. Ou C, Presthus J, Beadle E. Laparoscopic bladder neck suspension using hernia mesh and surgical staples. *J Laparoendosc Surg* 1993;3:563–6

30. Nezhat CH, Nezhat F, Nezhat CR, Rottenberg H. Laparoscopic retropubic cystourethropexy. *J Am Assoc Gynecol Laparosc* 1994;1:339–49

31. Nezhat CH, Nezhat F, Seidman DS, et al. A new method for laparoscopic access to the space of Retzius during retropubic cystourethropexy. *J Urol* 1996;155:1916–8

32. Richardson AC. How to correct prolapse paravaginally. *Comtemp Obstet Gynecol* 1990; 35(9):100–14

33. Weber AM, Walters MD. Anterior vaginal prolapse: Review of anatomy and techniques of surgical repair. *Obstet Gynecol* 1997;89: 311–8

34. Richardson AC, Lyon JB, Williams NL. A new look at pelvic relaxation. *Am J Obstet Gynecol* 1976;126:568–73

35. Richardson AC, Lyon JB, Williams NL. Treatment of stress urinary incontinence due to paravaginal fascial defect. *Obstet Gynecol* 1981;57:357–62

36. Baden WF, Walker TA. Urinary stress incontinence: Evolution of paravaginal repair. *Female Patient* 1987;12:89–94

37. Liu CY. Laparoscopic cystocele repair: Paravaginal suspension. In Liu CY, ed. *Laparoscopic Hysterectomy and Pelvic Floor Reconstruction.* Cambridge, MA: Blackwell Science, 1996:330–40

38. Dunton JD, Mikuta J. Post-hysterectomy vaginal vault prolapse. *Postgrad Obstet Gynecol* 1988;8:1–6

39. Sze EH, Miklos JR, Partoll L, *et al.* Sacrospinous ligament fixation with transvaginal needle suspension for advanced pelvic organ prolapse and stress incontinence. *Obstet Gynecol* 1997;89:129–32

40. Arthur HG, Savage D. Uterine prolapse and prolapse of vaginal vault treated by sacral hysteropexy. *J Obstet Gynaecol Br Emp* 1957; 64:355–60

41. Randall CL, Nichols DH. Surgical treatment of vaginal inversion. *Obstet Gynecol* 1971;38: 327–32

42. Symmonds RE, Williams TJ, Lee RA, Webb MJ. Post-hysterectomy enterocele and vaginal vault prolapse. *Am J Obstet Gynecol* 1981;140:852–9

43. Nezhat CH, Nezhat FR, Nezhat CR. Laparoscopic sacral colpopexy for vaginal vault prolapse. *Obstet Gynecol* 1994;84:885–8

16 Intravenous and local anesthesia

Raymond Glassenberg and Samuel Glassenberg

Monitoring of ventilation

When a patient is rendered unconscious by use of a potent inhalational agent or high dose of narcotic, or is merely sedated or awake and about to undergo surgery under local or regional anesthesia, the physiological functions which maintain life must be monitored. Respiratory rate can simply be counted by a trained observer. Adequacy of ventilation can be measured by monitoring the amount of exhaled carbon dioxide (CO_2) using a capnograph. This device samples exhaled gas for CO_2 by measuring the infrared absorption of CO_2 at specific wavelengths. At rest, the body produces 180 mL / min of CO_2, which is normally carried in the blood as bicarbonate 2.4 mEq / 100 mL of blood. If the bicarbonate were converted to

a gas, it would occupy a volume of 60 mL; therefore, a CO_2 content of 60 vol% is equivalent to 60 mL of CO_2 / 100 mL of blood. Thus,

$$PV = nRT \text{ wherein}$$
$$V = 0.0024 \times 0.082 \times (273 + 36) / 1 \text{ atm.}$$

During normal breathing, CO_2 is exhaled. The relationship between alveolar CO_2 partial pressure (PCO_2) and alveolar ventilation is given by the formula wherein

$$\text{alveolar } PCO_2 = 713 \text{ mmHg} \times$$
$$(CO_2 \text{ output} / \text{alveolar ventilation}).$$

If a patient is oversedated and the ventilatory rate falls, but the CO_2 production remains constant at 180 mL / min, then CO_2 will accumulate in the lungs and the alveolar PCO_2 will rise (Figure 16.1). Thus, if alveolar ventilation drops by half, from

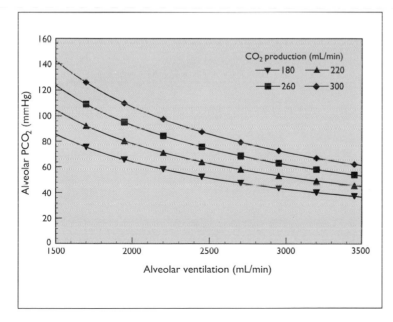

Figure 16.1 Plot of alveolar $PCO_2 = 713$ mmHg $\times$ (CO_2 output / alveolar ventilation). For the same level of ventilation, a faster rate of CO_2 production yields a higher alveolar PCO_2. Alveolar ventilation at 2100 mL / min and a CO_2 production at 180 mL / min produces the same alveolar PCO_2 as CO_2 production at 300 mL / min with an alveolar rate at 3500 mL / min

3500 to 1750 mL / min, the alveolar PCO_2 will rise to 72 mmHg.

During laparoscopy, the volume of CO_2 absorbed from the peritoneal cavity ranges from 18–40 mL / min[1-4]. This is usually not a problem if the patient is receiving a general anesthetic and ventilation is increased by a mechanical ventilator. However, the combination of heavy sedation with laparoscopy under local anesthesia can be dangerous. During laparoscopy when CO_2 production increases by 30% due to CO_2 absorption, if the alveolar ventilation falls to 1750 mL / min due to heavy sedation, the alveolar PCO_2 is likely to exceed 100 mmHg (see Figure 16.1), leading to arrhythmias and cardiac arrest. Laparoscopy performed under epidural anesthesia in the absence of sedation to blunt the respiratory centers is accompanied by a spontaneous 30% increase in alveolar ventilation and a normal alveolar PCO_2[5].

Monitoring of oxygenation

Adequacy of oxygenation can be measured with a pulse oximeter to measure oxygen saturation. This device measures the intensity of two different wavelengths of light transmitted through an arterial bed in a fingernail. With hemoglobin at 15 g / 100 mL and 100% saturation, arterial blood will contain 20 mL of oxygen / 100 mL of blood; thus,

$$\text{oxygen content} = (1.34 \times 15\,g \times 100\%\text{ saturation}).$$

Venous blood is only 75% saturated and therefore contains only 15 mL of oxygen / 100 mL of blood. Venous blood carries four times as much CO_2 (60 mL of CO_2 / 100 mL of blood) as it does oxygen (15 mL / 100 mL of blood). The difference between arterial and venous oxygen content is 5 vol%. This number multiplied by the average cardiac

output of 5000 mL / min gives an oxygen consumption of 250 mL / min.

If ventilation is inadequate, then not enough oxygen reaches the bloodstream through the lungs and the arterial oxygen saturation will fall. During normal breathing, oxygen enters the alveoli during inspiration. The relationship between alveolar oxygen partial pressure (PO_2) and alveolar ventilation is detailed by the formula wherein

$$\text{alveolar } PO_2 = 713\text{ mmHg} \times (\text{inspired } O_2 \text{ concentration} - O_2 \text{ uptake / alveolar ventilation})[6].$$

If a patient is oversedated and the ventilatory rate falls, but the oxygen uptake remains constant at 225 mL / min, then oxygen is removed from the lungs faster than it is replaced so that the alveolar PO_2 will fall. Thus, if alveolar ventilation drops from 3500 to 1750 mL / min, then alveolar PO_2 will fall to 60 mmHg.

The difference between alveolar and arterial PO_2 can vary from 10–35 mmHg. Alveolar hypoventilation can be detected by measuring arterial PO_2 (PaO_2) using a pulse oximeter. Hemoglobin oxygen saturation is related to PaO_2 by the formula wherein

$$\text{hemoglobin oxygen saturation} = (0.00013\,PO_2^{2.7}) / (1 + 0.00013\,PO_2^{2.7}).$$

Whereas hypoxemia due to hypoventilation can be treated by increasing the inspired oxygen concentration (Figure 16.2), this will do nothing to prevent the rise in alveolar PCO_2. The time course for the rise in alveolar PCO_2 following a decrease in ventilation during oxygen supplementation is shown in Figures 16.3 and 16.4[7]. If the alveolar ventilation is decreased to 1200 mL / min, the alveolar PCO_2 will double over 10 min whereas arterial saturation will hover around 90%. If the ventilation is decreased by 75% to 800 mL / min, then, within 10 min, the

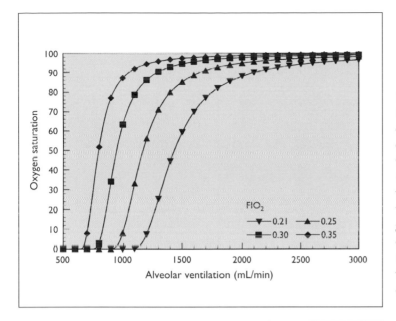

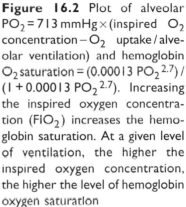

Figure 16.2 Plot of alveolar $PO_2 = 713$ mmHg $\times$ (inspired O_2 concentration $- O_2$ uptake / alveolar ventilation) and hemoglobin O_2 saturation $= (0.00013\ PO_2^{2.7}) / (1 + 0.00013\ PO_2^{2.7})$. Increasing the inspired oxygen concentration (FIO_2) increases the hemoglobin saturation. At a given level of ventilation, the higher the inspired oxygen concentration, the higher the level of hemoglobin oxygen saturation

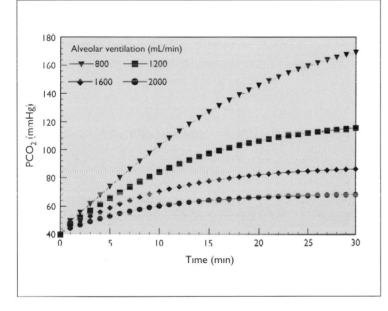

Figure 16.3 Plot showing the exponential relationship wherein the alveolar PCO_2 rises towards a limiting value as time increases and ventilation decreases

alveolar PCO_2 will be 100 mmHg and oxygen saturation will be 55%. Hypercarbia and hypertension are associated with cardiac arrhythmias in patients given oxygen supplementation[8].

The use of CO_2 for insufflation of the abdomen during gynecological procedures with the patient in a head-down position causes a 25% increase in mean arterial blood pressure, a 15% decrease in cardiac output and a 50% increase in systemic vascular resistance[9]. Some of these hemodynamic changes can be monitored by measuring blood pressure. However, intraoperative monitoring with capnography and pulse oximetry provide little information on the increase in vascular resistance and reduction in cardiac output except in

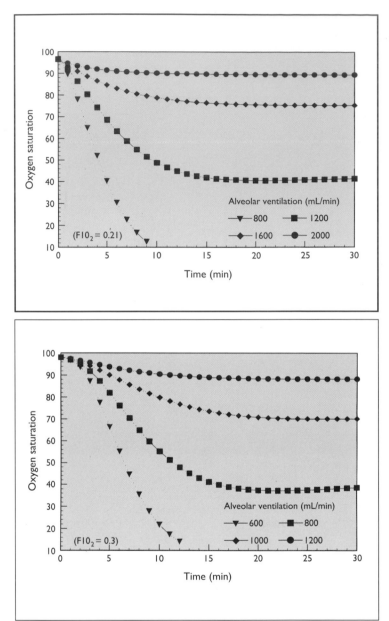

Figure 16.4 Plots showing the exponential relationship wherein hemoglobin oxygen saturation falls when ventilation is decreased (upper) and the protective effect of increasing the inspired oxygen concentration during hypoventilation when comparing oxygen saturation with alveolar ventilation at 1200 mL / min (lower)

special circumstances. A sudden drop in cardiac output can occur due to inadequate venous return or severe bradycardia. In such circumstances, not enough blood carrying CO_2 reaches the lungs, and the alveolar PCO_2 will decrease. A fall in alveolar PCO_2 can also occur if the patient suddenly develops an air or thombotic embolus. If the embolus is massive, then not enough blood is able to reach the ventilated alveoli and, thus, alveolar CO_2 and arterial oxygen saturation will both fall whereas the arterial PCO_2 will rise.

Indeed, during operative hysteroscopy, the phenomenon of oxygen desaturation accompanied by a simultaneous decrease in alveolar PCO_2 and increase in arterial PCO_2 has been observed, and attributed to an air embolism during endometrial resection[10].

Desaturation of arterial oxygen associated with hyponatremia can occur during hysteroscopy when large amounts of hypotonic solution are absorbed through open venous sinuses[11]. Thus, monitoring oxygen saturation and exhaled CO_2 can produce valuable information concerning cardiac output, pulmonary perfusion and adequacy of ventilation.

Intravenous medication

Conscious sedation is defined as "a minimally depressed level of consciousness that retains the patient's ability to maintain the airway independently and continuously and to respond appropriately to physical stimulation and verbal command." The drugs administered intravenously to provide conscious sedation are the same as those used to produce general anesthesia (Table 16.1). Depending on the size of the dose,

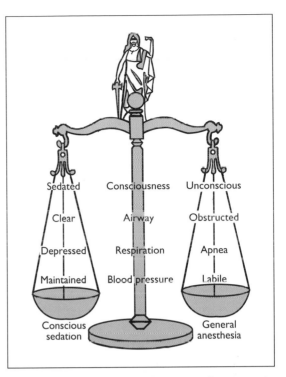

Figure 16.5 There is little margin for error in anesthesia

Table 16.1 Doses of intravenous sedative and analgesic drugs

	Dose	
	Conscious sedation	*General anesthesia*
Analgesics		
Alfentanil	0.5–1.0 mg	100–200 µg/kg
Butorphanol	1–2 mg	NA
Fentanyl	50–150 µg	50–150 µg/kg
Hydromorphone	0.5 2.0 mg	NA
Meperidine hydrochloride	30–100 mg	NA
Morphine sulfate	3–10 mg	1–5 mg/kg
Nalbuphine hydrochloride	5–15 mg	NA
Sufentanil	5–15 µg	5–20 µg/kg
Sedative/anxiolytic		
Diazepam	5–15 mg	—
Hydroxyzine	25–100 mg	—
Lorazepam	1–2 mg	—
Midazolam	2.5–7.5 mg	—
Propofol	25–50 mg	2 mg/kg
Thiopental	50–100 mg	4 mg/kg

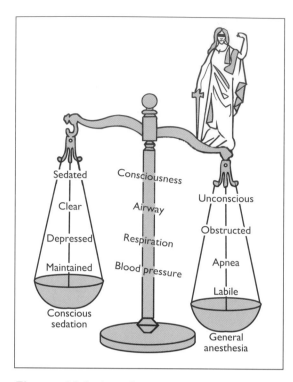

Figure 16.6 Anesthesia cannot be administered blindly; the patient must be monitored at all times

these drugs produce effects that range from minimal sedation to complete loss of consciousness, airway obstruction and apnea (Figure 16.5). The effects are also dependent on the patient's age, physical condition and genetic factors that affect drug metabolism.

These drugs should be administered in the presence of equipment that can provide ventilatory support. If too much drug is given, the patient's respiratory balance may be easily upset (Figure 16.6). There have been over 50 reports of respiratory or cardiac arrest in patients receiving a particular benzodiazepine for sedation during endoscopy because of inadequate monitoring[12].

During general anesthesia, recovery from an infusion of propofol is four times faster than that with midazolam. Patients receiving narcotic infusions for less than 3 h recover much more slowly with fentanyl than with sufentanil or alfentanil[13]. Both alfentanil and sufentanil are the drugs of choice for infusions of opioids lasting longer than 4 h (Figures 16.7 and 16.8). A

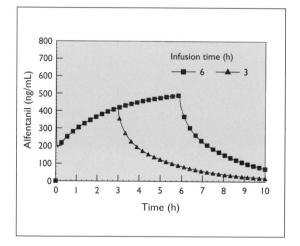

Figure 16.7 Computer simulation of plasma alfentanil concentration based on a 25 μg/kg bolus followed by a constant infusion of 1.5 μg/kg/min. The patient will not be able to breathe spontaneously until the plasma level falls below 100 ng/mL

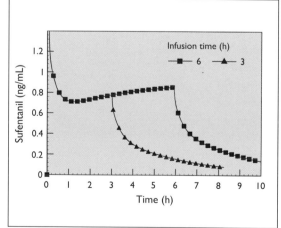

Figure 16.8 Computer simulation of plasma sufentanil concentration based on a 1 μg/kg bolus followed by a constant infusion of 0.8 μg/kg/min. The patient will not be able to breathe spontaneously until the plasma level falls below 0.25 ng/mL

narcotic-based anesthetic will require, even for short operations, at least 1 h from the time of termination of the infusion before the plasma concentration falls to a level adequate for spontaneous ventilation on awakening.

Local anesthetics

Local anesthetics work by blocking sodium channels in neural tissue, including peripheral neurons (peripheral nerve blocks), the spinal cord (spinal anesthesia), the heart

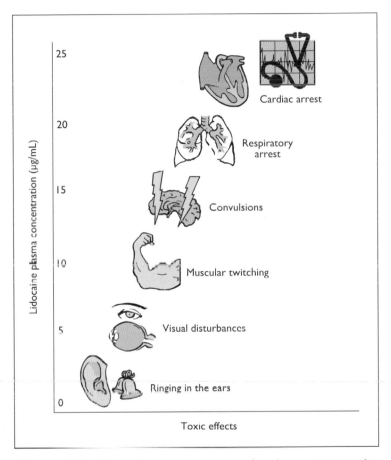

Figure 16.9 The dire consequences of a large intravascular injection of lidocaine

Table 16.2 Doses of local anesthetics and resultant blood levels

	Epidural dose	Blood level ($\mu g/mL$)	CNS toxicity ($\mu g/mL$)	Cardiac toxicity ($\mu g/mL$)
Chloroprocaine	400 mg		...	...
Lidocaine	400 mg	4	20	25
Mepivacaine	400 mg	4	22	—
Bupivacaine	200 mg	2	4–5	6

CNS, central nervous system

(lidocaine infusions to control ventricular arrhythmias) and the brain (where toxic levels can cause convulsions). When performing an epidural block using 200 mg of bupivacaine or 400 mg of lidocaine, care must be taken to ensure that the drug is appropriately placed. A systemic blood level of $1\,\mu g\,/\,mL$ is achieved for every 100 mg of drug deposited in the epidural space (Table 16.2).

A 400-mg bolus of lidocaine inadvertently injected into the vascular system will produce a blood level of $20–30\,\mu g\,/\,mL$, which is enough to cause seizures and respiratory arrest (Figure 16.9)[14]. Intravenous thiopental, diazepam or midazolam must then be given to terminate seizure

activity and intubation of the trachea may be necessary to restore ventilation.

Initially, bupivacaine was thought to be safer than lidocaine to use in obstetric cases because of its associated lower drug concentration in the umbilical cord compared with levels in maternal plasma. However, it is now known that neonatal plasma is deficient in $alpha_1$-acid glycoprotein to which bupivacaine binds, thus explaining the lower cord plasma concentration[15]. Bupivacaine occurs in solution as two isomers; the R form results in a fourfold greater decrease in cardiac conduction than seen with lidocaine. Ropivacaine, a new local anesthetic, is manufactured only as the S form and promises to be less cardiotoxic.

References

1. Puri GD, Singh H. Ventilatory effects of laparoscopy under general anaesthesia. *Br J Anaesth* 1992;68:211–3

2. Mullet CE, Viale JP, Sagnard PE, *et al.* Pulmonary CO_2 elimination during surgical procedures using intra- or extraperitoneal CO_2 insufflation. *Anesth Analg* 1993;7:622–6

3. Hirvonen EA, Nuutinen LS, Kauko M. Ventilatory effects, blood gas changes, and oxygen consumption during laparoscopic hysterectomy. *Anesth Analg* 1995;80:961–6

4. Tan PI, Lee TI, Tweed WA. Carbon dioxide absorption and gas exchange during pelvic laparoscopy. *Can J Anaesth* 1992;39:677–81

5. Ciofolo MJ, Clergue F, Seebacher J, *et al.* Ventilatory effects of laparoscopy under epidural anesthesia. *Anesth Analg* 1990;70:357–61

6. Nunn JF. *Applied Respiratory Physiology.* London: Butterworth & Co., 1977

7. Farmery AD, Roe PG. A model to describe the rate of oxyhaemoglobin desaturation during apnoea. *Br J Anaesth* 1996;76:284–91

8. Council on Scientific Affairs of the American Medical Association. The use of pulse oximetry during conscious sedation. *J Am Med Assoc* 1993;270:1463–8

9. Joris JL, Noirot DP, Legrand MJ, *et al.* Hemodynamic changes during laparoscopic cholecystectomy. *Anesth Analg* 1993;76:1067–71

10. Goldenberg M, Zolti M, Seidman DS, *et al.* Transient blood oxygen desaturation, hypercapnia, and coagulopathy after operative hysteroscopy with glycine used as the distending medium. *Am J Obstet Gynecol* 1994;1:25–9

11. Witz CA, Silverberg KM, Burns WN, *et al.* Complications associated with the absorption of hysteroscopic fluid media. *Fertil Steril* 1993;60:745–56

12. Food and Drug Administration. Warning re-emphasized in midazolam labeling. *FDA Drug Bull* 1986;27:5

13. Shafer SL, Varvel JR. Pharmacokinetics, pharmacodynamics, and rational opioid selection. *Anesthesiology* 1991;74:53–63

14. Tucker GT. Safety in numbers: The role of pharmacokinetics in local anesthetic toxicity. The 1993 ASRA lecture. *Reg Anesth* 1994; 19(3):155–63

15. Reynolds F. In defense of bupivacaine. *Int J Obstet Anesth* 1995;4:93–108

Selected bibliography

Myomectomy

Gutmann JN, Thornton K, Carcangiu M, Diamond MP. Evaluation of leuprolide acetate (LA) treatment on histopathology of uterine myomata. *Fertil Steril* 1994;61:622–6

LaMorte AL, Lalwani S, Diamond MP. Morbidity associated with abdominal myomectomy. *Obstet Gynecol* 1993;82:897–900

Meyer WR, Mayer AR, Diamond MP, *et al.* Unsuspected leiomyosarcoma: Treatment with a gonadotropin-releasing hormone analogue. *Obstet Gynecol* 1990;75:529–32

Schwartz LB, Diamond MP, Schwartz PE. Leiomyosarcomas: Clinical presentation. *Am J Obstet Gynecol* 1993;168:180–3

Endometriosis

Adamson D, Martin D, eds. *An Atlas of Endoscopic Management of Gynecologic Disease.* Philadelphia: Lippincott–Raven, 1996

Azziz R, Murphy A. *A Practical Manual of Operative Laparoscopy and Hysteroscopy.* New York: Springer-Verlag, 1997

Corfman R, Diamond MP, DeCherney AH, eds. *Complications of Laparoscopy and Hysteroscopy,* 2nd edn. Boston: Blackwell Scientific Publications, 1997

Diamond MP, Daniell JF, Jones HW III, eds. *Hysterectomy.* Boston: Blackwell Scientific Publications, 1995

Diamond MP, DeCherney AH, consult. eds, Johns DA, ed. Controversies in endoscopy. *Infertility and Reproductive Medicine Clinics of North America.* Philadelphia: WB Saunders, 1993;4: issue 2

Diamond MP, DeCherney AH, consult. eds, Phipps JH, ed. Adnexal masses. *Infertility and Reproductive Medicine Clinics of North America.* Philadelphia: WB Saunders, 1995;6: issue 3

Sanfilippo J, Levine R, eds. *Operative Gynecologic Endoscopy.* New York: Springer-Verlag, 1997

Sciarra JJ, ed. *Gynecology and Obstetrics.* Philadelphia: Harper & Row, 1996

Soderstrom R, ed. *Operative Laparoscopy: The Master's Techniques.* Philadelphia: Lippincott–Raven, 1997.

Sutton C, Diamond MP, eds. *Endoscopic Surgery for Gynaecologists,* 2nd edn. London: WB Saunders, 1997

Laparoscopically assisted vaginal hysterectomy

Johns DA, Diamond MP. Adequacy of laparoscopic oophorectomy. *J Am Assoc Gynecol Laparosc* 1993;1:20–3

Johns DA, Diamond MP. Laparoscopically assisted vaginal hysterectomles. *J Reprod Med* 1994; 39:424–8

Mage G, Bruhat M-A. Pregnancy following salpingostomy: Comparison between CO_2 laser and electrosurgery procedures. *Fertil Steril* 1983; 40:472–9

Pouly JL, Mahnes H, Mage G, Bruhat M. Conservative laparoscopic treatment of 321 ectopic pregnancies. *Fertil Steril* 1986;16: 1093–9

Ransom SB, White C, McNeeley SG, Diamond MP. A cost effectiveness evaluation of laparoscopic disposable versus nondisposable intraumbilical trocars. *J Am Assoc Gynecol Laparosc* 1996;4:25–8

Reich H, Johns DA, Davis G, Diamond MP. Laparoscopic oophorectomy. *J Reprod Med* 1993; 38:497–501

Russell JB, DeCherney AH, Laufer N, *et al.* Neosalpingostomy: A comparison of 24- and 72-month follow-up times show increased pregnancy rate. *Fertil Steril* 1986;45:296–301

Tulandi T. Salpingo-ovariolysis: A comparison between laser surgery and electrosurgery. *Fertil Steril* 1986;45:489–93

General reading

Daniell JF, Diamond MP, McLaughlin DS, *et al.* Clinical result of terminal salpingostomy using the CO_2 laser: Report of the Intra-Abdominal Laser Study Group. *Fertil Steril* 1986;45:175–8

DeCherney AH. The leader of the band is tired ... *Fertil Steril* 1985;44:299

Diamond MP. Surgical aspects of infertility. In Sciarra JJ, ed. *Gynecology and Obstetrics, Vol 5.* Philadelphia: Harper & Row, 1995

Diamond MP, Daniell JF, Feste J, *et al.* Adhesion reformation and *de novo* adhesion formation following reproductive pelvic surgery. *Fertil Steril* 1987;47:864–6

Diamond MP, Daniell JD, Feste J, *et al.* Initial report of the Carbon Dioxide Laser Laparoscopy Study Group: Complications. *J Gynecol Surg* 1989;5:269–72

Diamond MP, Daniell JF, Johns DA, *et al.* Postoperative adhesion development following operative laparoscopy: Evaluation at early second-look procedures. *Fertil Steril* 1991;55: 700–4

Diamond MP, Daniell JF, Martin DC, *et al.* Tubal patency and pelvic adhesions at early second look laparoscopy following intra-abdominal use of the carbon dioxide laser: Initial report of the Intra-Abdominal Laser Study Group. *Fertil Steril* 1984;42:717

Diamond MP, DeCherney AH. Distal segment tubal ectopic pregnancy after segmental resection of an isthmic ectopic. *J Reprod Med* 1988;33:236–7

Diamond MP, DeCherney AH, Polan ML. Laparoscopic use of the argon laser in non-endometriotic reproductive pelvic surgery. *J Reprod Med* 1986;31:1011–3

Diamond MP, Johns DA. Endometriosis. In Ballantyne G, Leahy P, Modlin IM, eds. *Laparoscopic Surgery.* Philadelphia: WB Saunders, 1994:379–94

Donnez J, Casanas-Roux F. Prognostic factors of fimbrial microsurgery. *Fertil Steril* 1986;46:200

Gomel V. Salpingo-ovariolysis by laparoscopy in infertility. *Fertil Steril* 1983;40:607

Goodman MP, Johns DA, Levine RL, *et al.* Report of the Study Group on Advanced Operative Laparoscopy (Pelviscopy). *J Gynecol Surg* 1989;5:353–60

Index